The Vagus Nerve in Therapeutic Practice

THE VAGUS NERVE IN THERAPEUTIC PRACTICE

Working with Clients to Manage Stress and Enhance Mind-Body Function

Ann Baldwin

Forewords by Dr. Rebecca Bailey and
Timothy G. Lohman, PhD

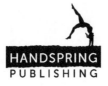

HANDSPRING
PUBLISHING

First published in Great Britain in 2024 by Handspring Publishing, an imprint of Jessica Kingsley Publishers
Part of John Murray Press

1

Disclaimer: The information contained in this book is not intended to replace the services of trained medical professionals or to be a substitute for medical advice. The complementary therapy described in this book may not be suitable for everyone to follow. You are advised to consult a doctor before embarking on any complementary therapy program and on any matters relating to your health, and in particular on any matters that may require diagnosis or medical attention.

A CIP catalogue record for this title is available from the British Library and the Library of Congress

ISBN 978 1 91342 655 2
eISBN 978 1 91342 656 9

Printed and bound in Great Britain by CPI Group, (UK) Ltd, Croydon CR0 4YY

Jessica Kingsley Publishers' policy is to use papers that are natural, renewable and recyclable products and made from wood grown in sustainable forests. The logging and manufacturing processes are expected to conform to the environmental regulations of the country of origin.

Handspring Publishing
Carmelite House
50 Victoria Embankment
London EC4Y 0DZ

www.handspringpublishing.com

John Murray Press
Part of Hodder & Stoughton Limited
An Hachette UK Company

Contents

Foreword

Dr. Baldwin's well-researched and informative book is a welcome addition to the growing understanding of somatic interventions. As a psychologist specializing in trauma, I have spent the last 25 years exploring what I later learned was the role of the vagal pathways in healing. My clinical practice was informed by my innate understanding of human nature, which from an early age was enhanced by my experience with horses. Incorporating horses into trauma treatment seemed to be a natural fit. Later, I learned horses were natural teachers in assisting clients in recognizing the nervous system's role in influencing human actions and reactions. For many clinicians, it was difficult to access the language and the scientific rationale to help communicate what they were seeing and experiencing. It turns out those of us who perceived themselves as far afield were, in fact, utilizing sound science by inadvertently choosing to incorporate the vagal pathways in our work. Laughing, chanting and equine interventions are validated by years of scientific research. The common denominator in these approaches is the amazing vagal nerve pathways. Dr. Baldwin helps fill in the blanks by masterfully weaving together the components that contribute to the healing power of down-regulating defense responses from a variety of modalities. Her book provides practitioners with much-needed sound explanations for what has been challenging to explain to skeptics and the uninformed.

The information offered by Dr. Baldwin helps the reader understand the nervous system's complexity and the fascinating dance between body and brain. When we operationalize trauma as a neural reaction to an event, as Dr. Porges' polyvagal theory requires, we are then faced with the challenge of helping "retune" the nervous system. Retuning the nervous system is, for most, unreachable through traditional talk therapy. The perspective that trauma is not about the physical insult but instead is the result of a dysregulated nervous system requires a multifaceted approach to treatment. Autonomic nervous system stabilization requires an adaptive nervous system; the nervous system's ability to flexibly tolerate and adapt to both stress and anxiety. A component of treatment is the promotion of the ability to tolerate physiological dysregulation in the service of achieving healthy homeostasis. It is a pursuit that requires the client's participation to effectively operationalize a shift in the nervous system's response patterns.

Trauma victims/survivors require careful treatment that considers their unique experiences and their individual nervous system responses. It is impossible to truly perceive how another person experiences the world around them. Helping a client understand their nervous system responses takes innovation, patience, presence and creativity. Dr. Baldwin has written a book that incorporates all three, as well as scientifically filling in the gaps to assist in explaining the how and the what behind the various interventions she presents. After reading this book, it becomes easier to explain the science behind their innovative practice. This book is an important contribution to a growing body of research on the power of the vagus nerve and to the overwhelming evidence that the mind-body connection is essential in trauma treatment.

Dr. Rebecca Bailey
Polyvagal Equine Institute
Co-founder of Connection-Focused Therapy with Linda Kohanov

To laugh a little is a start. To laugh a lot is a new beginning. ~ *Dr. B*

Foreword

It is unusual for a scientist and a clinician to write a book from both the perspectives of a clinician's skills and a researcher's mind. Dr. Ann Baldwin has done just that with her description of the vagus nerve and its many influences on the body. If you are a clinician interested in how certain practices can stimulate the vagus nerve affecting emotional stress, inflammation and heart rate variability (HRV), you will find this book of great use in your work. If you are curious, like me, about the role of the vagus nerve and the research that demonstrates its role in restoring health and wellness, you will gain a better understanding of the vagus nerve in therapeutic practices as well as your personal health.

Much of this book addresses ways to stimulate the vagus nerve in breathing, chanting, laughter and emotional participation. Clinical treatments of acupuncture, aromatherapy and massage, and how they influence vagal tone and lead to a healthier autonomic nervous system, are presented with empirical findings for their effectiveness.

In writing this book, Ann combines the skills of both disciplines, so that you as a reader or clinician can gain the benefit of a well-researched clinical practitioner. I first met Ann in one of her workshops while we both were professors in the Department of Physiology at the University of Arizona. Attending her workshops on Reiki and on HRV and heart health, I was immediately struck by her ability to evaluate and explain physiological effects from a clinical perspective.

In two of my favorite chapters, I learned about HRV and breath control and about Equine Assisted Learning (EAL). The easiest way to increase HRV is to breathe more slowly and deeply than usual. There is a lot to learn about increasing the activity of the vagus nerve and HRV, how it works and the effects of increased HRV and your heart health.

With EAL, the book explores how vagal stimulation enhances your relationship with others. Equine Assisted Learning brings you into the horse's world where a horse–human interaction is experienced, while standing on the ground. How horses respond to you and how you respond to a horse can lead to regulation of your autonomic nervous system with a qualified EAL facilitator. Ann is that kind of guide, and an experienced guide is crucial to a successful horse meeting. Scientific studies monitoring physiological changes in both you and the horse have been well documented. Ann reports that for those who have been traumatized, deep breathing, gently stroking the horse and rocking back and forth will allow the person to experience a healing relationship and moments when they become "horse whisperers," as the patient and the horse help each other.

There are outstanding case histories in each chapter to illustrate the practical methods used to stimulate the vagal complex and restore the autonomic nervous system to a healthy level. In one case, Ann describes a woman who is a top-level manager with a low-level baseline HRV, a heart rate which varied in time in a random pattern and a low-level of coherence with her sympathetic and parasympathetic systems. In five sessions, this woman learned to change her breathing pattern, her thoughts and bring into balance her sympathetic and parasympathetic function.

The Vagus Nerve in Therapeutic Practice is a well-written and unusual book combining the science behind many clinical treatments for the benefit of the practitioner. In this fast-paced world, Dr. Baldwin offers essential information to help all of us better adapt and I highly recommend it.

Timothy G. Lohman, PhD
Professor Emeritus
The University of Arizona

Acknowledgments

I would like to thank my physiology undergraduate students at the University of Arizona who took my course "Physiology of Mind-Body Interactions" and whose enthusiasm and feedback made me realize how important it was to them to be able to access their vagus nerve.

I am also grateful to my clients at Mind-Body-Science for giving me the chance to help them with various physical, mental and emotional imbalances and for providing me with some wonderful stories about how they used the mind-body techniques to improve their lives.

Preface

Up until 2008, I was a tenured Professor of Physiology at the University of Arizona. Around the year 2000, my research direction changed, and I started to become interested in how mental and emotional stress deleteriously affect the body. I was also searching for effective solutions to this problem and set up experiments to test the effectiveness of therapies such as Reiki, biofeedback, listening to live harp music, equine-assisted learning, and yoga. The results of these experiments were a turning point in my career. I took the huge step of giving up my full-time tenured position at the University of Arizona so that I could devote time to helping people reduce their stress with biofeedback and Reiki. I started my business, Mind-Body-Science, and continued part-time at the University of Arizona as an active researcher.

After a few years of treating mostly middle-aged people, it occurred to me that young people really needed to learn these techniques so they could improve their physical health, cognitive skills and emotional regulation early on. I put together an undergraduate class called "Physiology of Mind-Body Interactions," one of the few physiology classes at the University of Arizona that focused on practical skills. The course was approved, and the students enrolled. They were highly motivated – most of them wanted to go to medical or dental school – and they quickly mastered the skills of autonomic regulation, especially activating the vagus nerve. As a result, they reaped the benefits.

Brittany said:

This class has been one of my favorites of all my years at the U of A and I will be incorporating the teachings into everyday life for as long as possible after I graduate!

Michelle said:

I gained a vast amount of knowledge and learned how daily-life activities and decisions affect our mind-body interactions and heart rate variability. As for my future, I know I will continue using the skills I gained from this class and applying them to my life.

Olivia said:

As a class, we persevered and navigated through the beginning of COVID in Spring of 2020, a feat whose difficulty should not be underestimated, and certainly one I will not forget. We all made good use of the breathing techniques you taught during that confusing time. I will always use these techniques to increase HRV, especially as I go through dental school these next few years.

As a scientist, educator and a provider of biofeedback and Reiki to people experiencing stress-related problems, I was delighted when Mary Law, then Director and Co-Owner of Handspring Publishing, asked me to write this book, *The Vagus Nerve in Therapeutic Practice.* I had not realized it, but based on my experiences with clients and students, this was a book that I needed to write. A book for people who are looking for non-invasive, inexpensive and effective ways to regain their autonomic balance by activating their vagus nerve so they can relax, digest, improve clarity of thought and socially engage. Practical, evidence-based methods are presented to stimulate the vagal complex, each illustrated by a case history from a complementary medicine or holistic practice. In this book, complementary medicine practitioners and holistic healers will discover ways to adapt their treatments so that their clients' experiences and outcomes are vastly improved.

My goal is to include accurate information about the anatomy and evolution of the vagus nerve, including how it communicates with the brain through the limbic system, and its possible role in promoting social engagement, as proposed in the polyvagal theory, but to keep the science light and understandable. The functions of the major branches of the vagus nerve and other neighboring cranial nerves are discussed in turn, each with a practical way to engage that specific nerve branch.

An addendum is included with charts that summarize the various exercises described throughout the book, as well as routines for utilizing combinations of the exercises on a daily, weekly and monthly basis. The book will enable healthcare professionals to attain a solid grasp of the clinical significance of regulating the vagus nerve and provide them with easy-to-follow ways to do it. If you have found other books on the vagus nerve to be, on the one hand, too technical, or, on the other hand, too simplified, this book is for you.

Ann Baldwin
Tucson, AZ, USA
December 2022

Glossary

Autonomic nervous system (ANS) The part of the nervous system responsible for control of bodily functions that are not consciously directed, such as breathing, the heartbeat and digestive processes. The autonomic nervous system is divided into **sympathetic** and **parasympathetic** fibers. Activation of sympathetic nerves increases arousal and heart rate whereas activation of parasympathetic nerves calms the mind and body for digestion, cellular maintenance and repair.

Cranial nerves A set of 12 nerves, including the vagus, that originate in the brain. Each has a different function responsible for sense or movement. Sensory cranial nerves help a person see, smell and hear. Conversely, motor cranial nerves help control muscle movements in the head and neck.

Heart rate variability (HRV) The second-by-second change in heart rate as a function of time that reflects the interaction between sympathetic and parasympathetic autonomic nervous system activity. High HRV is associated with optimal mind-body function and adaptability. Low HRV is associated with states of physical, mental and emotional stress.

Interoception The collection of senses perceiving the internal state of the body. It is the sense that allows us to answer the question "How do I feel?" in any given moment.

Limbic system A collection of brain structures that integrate the various bodily sensations, thoughts and memories experienced or recalled at a particular moment into a complex electrical signal.

Microbiome The collection of bacteria, fungi, viruses, and their genes, that naturally live on the inner surface of the gut. It can influence signals sent from nerve endings in the intestine to the brain via the vagus nerve and can affect mood. Likewise, thoughts and emotions can affect the composition of the microbiome.

Polyvagal theory The theory that proposes three evolutionary stages of the ANS, the latest being the "ventral vagal complex" that rapidly regulates cardiac output to foster engagement, and recruits cranial nerves to facilitate facial expressions and vocalization required for social behaviors.

Respiratory sinus arrythmia This occurs when a person's heart rate associates with their breathing cycle such that when they breathe in, their heart rate increases, and when they breathe out, their heart rate decreases. Typically, its presence is an indicator of good cardiovascular health.

Vagus nerve A nerve that supplies nerve fibers to the pharynx (throat), larynx (voice box), trachea (windpipe), lungs, heart, esophagus and intestinal tract, and interfaces with the parasympathetic control of the heart. The vagus nerve also brings sensory information back to the brain from the ear, tongue, pharynx, larynx, heart and intestine.

Importance of Self-Regulating the Autonomic Nervous System

The mind and body communicate through two systems: the autonomic nervous system (ANS) which automatically regulates the functions of organs and glands without any need for conscious control, and the endocrine system which releases hormones from the glands to optimize mind-body function under a wide variety of conditions. This book will be concerned mainly with the ANS because its focus is the vagus nerve, which, with its cranial and sacral branches, makes up the parasympathetic portion of the ANS. However, since one function of the ANS is to stimulate the glands to produce hormones, the roles of the endocrine system will be incorporated into the discussion in these instances.

The vagus nerve is the longest nerve in the ANS and its name is Latin for "wanderer." There are, in fact, two vagus nerves, left and right, but they are typically referred to collectively as a single system. The vagus nerve has many branches that serve various body organs and structures. In addition, the vagus nerve works in conjunction with 11 other cranial nerves serving the head, facial and neck areas, and five sacral nerves serving the lower body including the bladder and genitals. Details of the other cranial nerves are given in Chapter 2. Discussion of the sacral nerve stimulation is not included in the book. These nerves regulate bladder and bowel function, which are not of concern here except for in colon hydrotherapy.

Although the ANS operates without conscious intervention, its function can be influenced by our thoughts and emotions. Thoughts and emotions consciously perceived in the mind alter sympathetic and parasympathetic activities. Autonomic function is also influenced by the way we breathe. As will be explained in Chapter 5, breath depth and frequency, as well as the time spent on each inhale versus each exhale, also affect the ANS. Long, deep breaths, with more time spent on the exhale than the inhale, signal our parasympathetic nervous system to calm the body down, whereas rapid, shallow chest breathing reduces parasympathetic, or vagal, activity.

NERVOUS SYSTEM

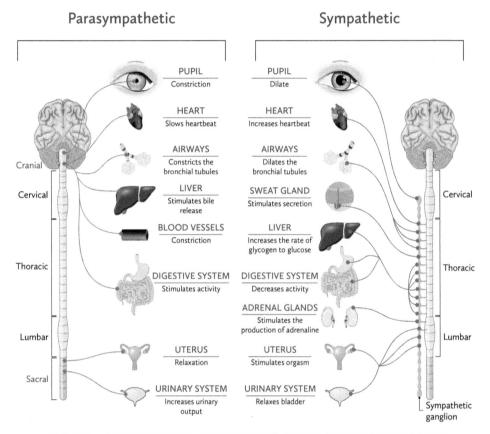

FIGURE I.1 ANATOMICAL DIFFERENCES IN PARASYMPATHETIC AND SYMPATHETIC DIVISIONS OF THE AUTONOMIC NERVOUS SYSTEM.

The use of breath and emotional perception to alter ANS function is called "self-regulation." Self-regulation is important because when we are under stress, the sympathetic component of the ANS, or "fight or flight response," takes over from the parasympathetic, or "rest and digest," component. This reaction is appropriate in the short term because it increases blood circulation so that more oxygen and nutrients can be delivered to the body, and it also elevates glucose concentration in the blood. These responses provide us with extra energy to help us resolve the stressful situation in the moment. However, if we are under chronic stress, caused by factors such as living in poverty, feeling undervalued, being forced to live by principles to which we are morally opposed, or trying to fulfil expectations that exceed our resources, the "fight or flight" responses are perpetuated over the long term and begin to drain the body's resources. As a result, we may become prone to digestive problems, headaches, muscle tension, sleep problems, weight gain, hypertension, heart disease, anxiety and depression.

The key to resolving these deleterious manifestations of chronic stress is to shift the ANS from "fight or flight" or sympathetic stimulation to "rest and digest" or parasympathetic stimulation. This latter response is dependent on the activity of the vagus nerve. Figure 1.1 depicts the parasympathetic and sympathetic components of the ANS and the organs that each branch serves.

WAYS TO STIMULATE THE VAGUS NERVE

So, how do we stimulate the vagus nerve and its associated branches as well as other cranial nerves (the vagal complex)? The purpose of this book is to answer that question by describing how various techniques related to breath regulation (such as heart-focused breathing, chanting, laughter yoga, aromatherapy), emotional perception (such as feeling gratitude, appreciating nature, bonding with a horse), direct or indirect touch (such as massage, acupuncture, colon hydrotherapy) or dietary manipulation can be used to stimulate the vagal complex. Examples will be given of specific therapies that utilize each of these techniques or combinations of techniques, and in many instances a case study will be included to illustrate these procedures as used in practice. Each technique will be linked to the anatomy of the vagal complex to demonstrate exactly which part of the vagal complex is being utilized in each case.

BRIEF ANATOMY OF THE VAGUS NERVE

A simple diagram showing the anatomy of the vagus nerve and how it connects to the brain and to the other major organs throughout the body is given in Figure 1.2. More details about the exact anatomical connections between the vagus nerve and the brain will be provided in Chapter 1.

The vagus nerve connects to the brain stem through the medulla oblongata which indirectly communicates with the limbic system (Figure 1.3), the part of the brain that deals with emotional processing. The limbic system and its various components will be discussed in more detail in Chapter 7.

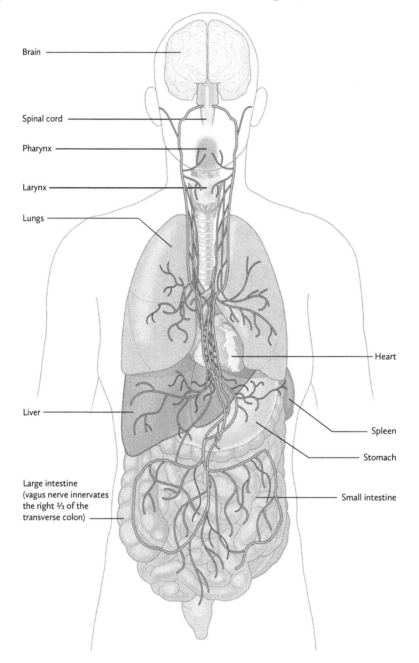

Brain

Spinal cord

Pharynx

Larynx

Lungs

Heart

Liver

Spleen

Stomach

Large intestine
(vagus nerve innervates
the right ⅔ of the
transverse colon)

Small intestine

FIGURE 1.2 ANATOMY OF THE VAGUS NERVE.

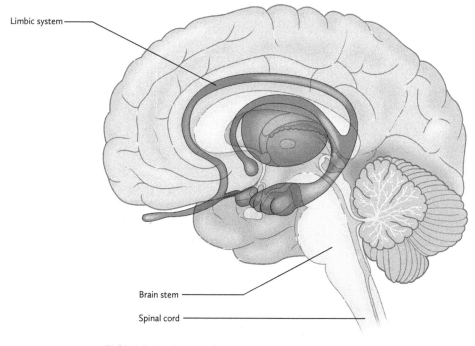

Limbic system

Brain stem

Spinal cord

FIGURE 1.3 BRAIN STEM AND LIMBIC SYSTEM.

THE IMPORTANCE OF THE LIMBIC SYSTEM

The vagus nerve transmits sensory information from the body through the brain stem, medulla oblongata and other associated structures to the limbic system. In addition, the vagus nerve is unique in that it carries both motor fibers and sensory fibers instead of just one type or the other. This means that directives for motor control, associated with the body's organs and structures, can also be transmitted through the vagus nerve from the brain to the body.

Apart from receiving sensory information from the body via the vagus nerve, the limbic system also acquires information from the prefrontal cortex, a part of the brain associated with cognition and decision making. So, the tight feeling in your stomach you experience as you wait for your medical test results has already been sent from your stomach through the limbic system to your prefrontal cortex, making you aware of the discomfort. Next, your decision to take a few deep breaths to relax yourself is communicated to the limbic system which then signals the ANS to shift from "fight or flight" mode to the "rest and digest" mode. In this way, the limbic system connects the mind and the body.

VAGAL FUNCTIONS

Two key roles of the vagus complex are to control the stress response by stimulating feelings of calm and relaxation and to facilitate digestion, by regulating movement of food through the intestine by peristalsis and by inducing the secretion of appropriate neurotransmitters and hormones to enable absorption of nutrients into the bloodstream. Figure 1.4 illustrates how some bodily functions are altered when nerves from the vagal complex are stimulated. Constricted pupils, enhanced salivation, reduced depth of breathing, slower heart rate, increased intestinal activity and urination are all consistent with the "rest and digest" response, relaxation, eating and digestion.

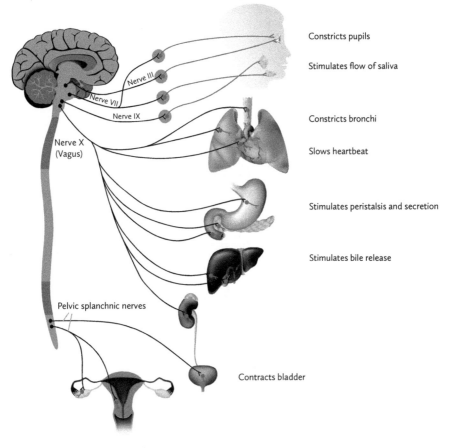

FIGURE 1.4 PARASYMPATHETIC SYSTEM.

However, according to the polyvagal theory (Porges 2003), the vagal complex does more than just regulate digestion and promote relaxation. Dorsal fibers in the back of the vagus nerve take care of those processes, but the *ventral* fibers in the front of the nerve appear to fine-tune how the heart rate varies with time (heart rate variability), allowing more frequent input to the heart rhythm from the vagal system. As described in Chapter 4, this makes the heart more able to adapt to constantly changing internal and external conditions, so its function is not locked into the "fight or flight" mode.

When the heart can respond readily to changing circumstances, the heart rate variability adopts a characteristic rhythm that is communicated through the ANS to the limbic system and then to the prefrontal cortex. The result is a shift to a calmer, more balanced mind-body state that is conducive to social engagement. In addition, the ventral vagus is neuroanatomically linked to the cranial nerves that promote social engagement via eye contact, facial expression and vocalization. This association of the vagus and other cranial nerves, termed the "ventral vagal complex," facilitates hearing, eating, speech, singing, nursing, kissing and smiling, which are all part of social engagement.

According to the polyvagal theory, the ANS consists of three evolutionary stages, the "dorsal vagus" which fosters digestion and responds to mental stress by depressing metabolic activity (the freeze response), the "sympathetic nervous system" which can increase metabolic output to foster mobilization behaviors necessary for the "fight or flight" response, and the "ventral vagal complex" which can rapidly regulate cardiac output to foster engagement and recruit cranial nerves that facilitate the facial expressions and vocalization required for social behaviors.

TECHNIQUES FOR ENHANCING VAGAL FUNCTIONS

In this book, we focus on how different parts of the vagal complex can be stimulated to perform their associated functions at will, and we recommend the types of therapy that can assist in each case. The 12 cranial nerves (I to XII) including the vagus nerve are listed below, together with their functions and some recommended therapies (in italics) designed to stimulate vagal tone in each case.

I. Olfactory nerve: smell – *aromatherapy.*

II. Optic nerve: carries visual information from retina to brain.

III. Oculomotor nerve: eye movement, constriction of pupil.

IV. Trochlear nerve: rotational movement of eye.

V. Trigeminal nerve: sensation and motor function of face and mouth – *laughter yoga, heart-focused breathing and stroking, social engagement.*

VI. Abducens nerve: lateral movement of eye.

VII. Facial nerve: face muscles, salivation – *laughter yoga, heart-focused breathing and stroking, social engagement.*

VIII. Vestibulocochlear or auditory nerve: carries sound from inner ear to brain.

IX. Glossopharyngeal nerve: swallowing and salivation.

X. Vagus nerves (left and right), commonly known as "the vagus nerve," which has the following branches:

- Pharyngeal: muscles of pharynx and soft palate – *swallowing*
- Laryngeal: vocal cords – *yogic chanting, heart-focused breathing and stroking, somatic therapy, social engagement*
- Auricular branch: carries sensory information to skin overlying external ear – *acupuncture*
- Inferior cervical cardiac branch: provides a parasympathetic connection to the heart and is key to regulating emotions – *forest bathing (walking in nature), biofeedback (gratitude), somatic therapy, heart-focused breathing and stroking, healing trauma with a horse (Rock-Back and Sigh)*
- Pulmonary branches: breathing, laughter – *laughter yoga, somatic therapy, massage and breathwork, heart-focused breathing and stroking, healing trauma with a horse (Rock-Back and Sigh)*
- Abdominal and intestinal branches: digestive system, microbiome – *colon hydrotherapy, acupuncture, diet and microbiome.*

XI. Spinal accessory nerve: movement of shoulders and neck – *massage and breathwork.*

XII. Hypoglossal nerve: tongue movement for speech – *heart-focused breathing and stroking, social engagement.*

In Chapter 2, we will consider the detailed functions of three cranial nerves – the auricular, olfactory and spinal accessory – and how they enhance vagal function when stimulated by acupuncture, aromatherapy and massage, respectively. The auricular branch carries sensory information to the skin overlying the ear and can be stimulated by acupuncture to calm the mind and provide pain relief. The olfactory branch regulates smell and can be activated by breathwork and aromatherapy to produce a relaxing effect. The spinal accessory nerve controls the movement of the shoulders and neck and can be stimulated using massage to provide pain relief.

In Chapter 3, we focus on the laryngeal branches of the vagus nerve which innervate the laryngeal muscles required for speaking, singing and chanting. When these nerves are stimulated – for example, by yogic chanting or laughter yoga – the body relaxes. The pulmonary branch of the vagus nerve also plays a major role in why these therapies are successful because attention to the breath is a key component of yogic chanting and laughter yoga.

As previously mentioned, emotions play a huge role in self-regulation of the vagal nerve, and they exert their influence through the heart. We have all experienced the thumping of our hearts when we spot a snake on the side of the path we are taking as we hike. Likewise, we notice how the thumping quickly abates when we realize it is a hose. Feeling fear and relief, like all emotions, affects the heart through the ANS. Fear stimulates the sympathetic nerves, whereas relief activates the inferior cervical cardiac branch of the vagus nerve which provides a parasympathetic connection to the heart. We will explore how emotions such as gratitude and appreciation activate the ventral vagal complex resulting in improved well-being in Chapter 4.

The way we breathe is also a key influencer of vagal stimulation and it acts through the pulmonary branches of the vagus nerve. The mechanisms by which breathing more deeply and slowly than usual produces feelings of calm and balance will be investigated in Chapter 5. Many types of therapies, such as massage, laughter yoga, somatic therapy and equine therapy include some breathwork, and therapists who are also accomplished in biofeedback can convincingly demonstrate visually to their clients how their breathing affects their heart rate variability in real time.

A key role of the vagus system is to facilitate digestion, and this is mediated through the abdominal and intestinal branches of the vagus nerve. So just eating a good meal will stimulate these parasympathetic nerves and shift you to a relaxed state, as described in Chapter 6. In a similar way, colon hydrotherapy can improve mood, by temporarily expanding the colon as occurs during peristalsis, and activating the stretch receptors in the colonic walls to stimulate the vagus system.

Diet can also influence mood. Recent research has revealed a fascinating connection between the microbiome – the collection of bacteria, fungi, viruses, and their genes, that naturally live on the inner surface of the gut – and mood. The composition of the microbiome is influenced by colonic irrigation and by diet. Changes in the microbiome and its metabolites are sensed by peripheral nerves in the inner lining of the intestine. These nerves may respond by stimulating the release of neurotransmitters and hormones, such as serotonin and dopamine, that are known to influence mood. The electrical signals these peripheral nerves send on to the vagus nerve and the limbic system respond to chemical changes in the gut. Since the amygdala is the part of the limbic system associated with emotional processes, its response to changes in the signal from the gut may affect mood. In Chapter 6, we will explore the link between diet and mood.

Chapter 7 will focus on the role played by the limbic system in self-regulating the vagal complex. It is thought that trauma can shock the ANS into a state of hyperarousal and hypervigilance or, in severe cases, into a freeze response. Hyperarousal is associated with an overactive amygdala, and the freeze response (hypoarousal) with an underactive amygdala. If the memory of the trauma remains unspeakable for too long, then the mental processing required for recovery cannot occur, and these states persist even when the person is not consciously thinking of the trauma.

Unresolved emotional trauma is often linked to bodily sensations such as pain, and it has been hypothesized that emotional trauma can reside in the body in the form of muscular tension. Since the mind and the body are intimately linked through the limbic system, it is possible that by using techniques to balance the ANS and release the tension in the body, the amygdala will rebalance and the emotional trauma will also dissipate. This is the theory behind somatic therapy in which physical stimuli such as touch, movement and breathwork are used to stimulate the vagal complex, promote feelings of relaxation and allow release of the physical and emotional tension associated with the trauma.

Finally, Chapter 8 presents Equine Assisted Learning (EAL), or guided interactions with horses, as an aid for honing the skills of self-regulation, particularly those related to breath control. Horses, as prey animals, are continually aware of their environment and provide instant feedback to humans regarding how they are behaving, their body language and the emotions they are feeling and emanating. A horse will usually respond more favorably to a person who breathes slowly and deeply, compared to one who, perhaps out of fear or anxiety, shows up with fast, shallow chest breathing. By tuning into their own physical sensations and emotions in the present moment, and observing how the horses respond to them, people can learn how to regulate their ANS, using vagal stimulation skills.

Our research has shown that when people are in a balanced autonomic state, which we call "relaxed alertness," horses are much more likely to engage and interact with them. Horses are large animals that can be unpredictable in their nature, and it is essential that this work is performed under the guidance of an equine professional and a facilitator. In this way, EAL provides a safe and secure opportunity for real-life practice of self-regulation skills as well as the possibility of forming social bonds with the horses and other participants.

REFERENCES

Porges SW, 2003. Social engagement and attachment. A phylogenetic perspective. *Ann N Y Acad Sci.* 1008: 31–47. doi: 10.1196/annals.1301.004.

CHAPTER 1

Anatomy and Evolution of the Vagus Nerve

In this chapter, we will start with the anatomy and function of the cranial nerves, of which the vagus nerve is one. The cranial nerves appear to work together as a system to facilitate relaxation and social engagement. One measurable influence of the vagus nerve on the heart is how it affects heart rate variability (HRV). This term will be defined and introduced early on because it is an important marker of stress and of vagal function. Then we will describe how the vagus nerve connects with the brain by means of the limbic system, which regulates communication between the brain and the body. Next, we will consider the uniqueness of the vagus nerve in that it contains both sensory and motor fibers, and that the motor fibers can be either dorsal (unmyelinated) or ventral (myelinated), equipping them for vastly different functions. Finally, we will present the "polyvagal theory" which is based on three evolutionary stages of the ANS and purports that the myelinated vagus is the most recently evolved stage which fosters engagement and disengagement with the environment.

ANATOMY AND FUNCTION OF THE CRANIAL NERVES

The vagus nerve and its branches form a major part of the parasympathetic nervous system (PNS). Acetylcholine (ACH), one of its major neurotransmitters, binds to immune cells and acts as an anti-inflammatory agent, and serotonin, another neurotransmitter (dubbed the "feel-good hormone"), is essential for the digestive process. The vagus nerve is the tenth of the 12 cranial nerves, is the longest nerve in the body and innervates all major organs in the body, hence its name, which is Latin for "wanderer." There are two sets of cranial nerves

(CN), and hence two vagal nerves, one on each side of the spine, but the pair is generally referred to as "the vagus nerve." A diagram of the arrangement of the vagus nerve (CN X) and some of the other cranial nerves (CN III, CN VII and CN IX) is shown in Figure 1.1. The three sacral or splanchnic nerves that control the genitals and bladder are also included in this diagram. Electrical stimulation of sacral nerves is used to control overactive bladders, but this issue will not be covered in this book.

The cranial nerves, attached to the brain, are primarily responsible for the sensory and motor functions of the head and neck. The exception is the vagus nerve. There are 12 cranial nerves, three of which are solely composed of sensory fibers, five are strictly motor fibers and the other four are mixed nerves. The first (olfactory), second (optic) and eighth (vestibulocochlear or auditory) nerves are purely sensory. The three nerves controlling eye movement – third (oculomotor), fourth (trochlear) and sixth (abducens) – are all motor, as are the eleventh (spinal accessory) and twelfth (hypoglossal). The remaining nerves, fifth (trigeminal), seventh (facial), ninth (glossopharyngeal), and tenth (vagus) contain both sensory and motor fibers.

The olfactory nerves (CN I) and optic nerves (CN II) emerge from the forebrain and the remaining ten pairs arise from various parts of the brain stem: the oculomotor (CN III) and trochlear (CN IV) nerves from the midbrain; the trigeminal nerve (CN V) from the pons; and the abducens (CN VI), facial (CN VII), auditory (CN VIII), glossopharyngeal (CN IX), vagus (CN X), spinal accessory (CN XI) and hypoglossal (CN XII) from the medulla oblongata. Table 1.1 shows the function of each of the 12 nerves and their central (brain stem) and peripheral (target muscle or ganglion – group of peripheral nerve cells) connections.

The functions and sensory/motor properties of the cranial nerves shown in Figure 1.1 are summarized as follows:

- Oculomotor (III): mixed cranial nerve responsible for eyeball movement, stimulates the lacrimal gland.
- Facial (VII): mixed cranial nerve, stimulates salivation.
- Glossopharyngeal (IX): mixed cranial nerve, involved in swallowing and salivation.
- Vagus (X): mixed cranial nerve, carries 80 percent of parasympathetic outflow to heart, airways, liver, gallbladder, stomach, small intestine and part of large intestine.

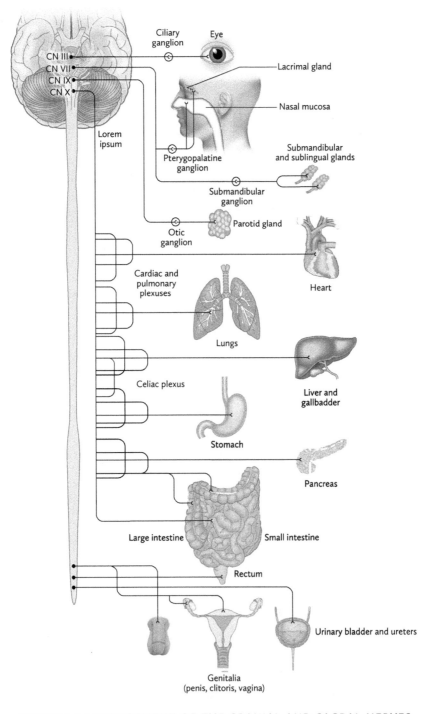

FIGURE 1.1 ARRANGEMENT OF THE CRANIAL AND SACRAL NERVES.
Source: Adapted from https://antranik.org/wp-content/uploads/2011/11/
parasympathetic-division-cranial-outflow-and-sacral-outflow.jpg.

Table 1.1 Cranial nerves

#	Name	Function (S, M or B)	Central connection	Peripheral connection
I	Olfactory	Smell (S)	Olfactory bulb (links to nucleus solitarius)	Olfactory epithelium
II	Optic	Vision (S)	Hypothalamus/thalamus/midbrain	Retina
III	Oculomotor	Eye movements (M)	Oculomotor nucleus	Extraocular muscles
IV	Trochlear	Rotational eye movements (M)	Trochlear nucleus	Superior oblique muscle
V	Trigeminal	Sensory/motor face (B)	Trigeminal nucleus	Trigeminal
VI	Abducens	Lateral eye movements (M)	Abducens nucleus	Lateral rectus muscle
VII	Facial	Motor: face, salivation Sensory: Taste (B)	Facial nucleus, nucleus solitarius, superior salivatory nucleus	Facial muscles, geniculate ganglion (taste)
VIII	Auditory	Hearing: carries sound from inner ear to brain Balance (S)	Cochlear nucleus, vestibular nucleus/cerebellum	Spiral ganglion (hearing), vestibular ganglion (balance)
IX	Glossopharyngeal	Motor: throat, swallowing, salivation Sensory: Taste (B)	Nucleus solitarius, inferior salivatory nucleus, nucleus ambiguus	Pharyngeal muscles, geniculate ganglion
X	Vagus	Motor/sensory: viscera (autonomic) (B)	Dorsal motor nucleus, nucleus ambiguus, nucleus solitarius	Ganglia serving heart and small intestine
XI	Spinal accessory	Motor: head, shoulders and neck (M)	Spinal accessory nucleus	Neck muscles
XII	Hypoglossal	Motor: lower throat, tongue – movement for speech (M)	Hypoglossal nucleus	Muscles of the larynx and lower pharynx

S, sensory; M, motor; B, both.

As shown in Figure 1.1, the vagus nerve (CN X) branches off to all major organs. The branches serving the larynx, lungs, heart and the intestines are listed in Table 1.2. They can easily be stimulated using various therapies in order to enhance vagal tone. These therapies and how they stimulate the various vagal nerve branches will be addressed in detail in later chapters.

Table 1.2 Therapies that stimulate each vagal branch

Vagal nerve branch	Yogic chant	Laughter yoga	Breath-work	Somatic therapy	EAL	Bio-feed-back	Colon hydro-therapy	Diet	Acu-puncture
Laryngeal	✓	✓		✓					
Pulmonary	✓	✓	✓	✓	✓	✓	✓		
Cardiac	✓	✓	✓	✓	✓	✓			
Intestinal							✓	✓	✓

Most of the 12 cranial nerves, including those shown in Figure 1.1, innervate organs, structures or glands that are necessary for social engagement. For example, movement of the eyeball is needed for making eye contact, facial nerves for showing facial expressions, and swallowing and salivation for eating, which often accompanies socialization. The vagus connection to the heart (inferior cardiac branch) also prepares the body for social interaction by providing a parasympathetic input to the heart through the ventral vagal fibers. In fact, if this input were absent, our heart rate would average about 100 beats per minute instead of the usual 60–80 beats per minute. The parasympathetic influence on the heart changes the frequency spectrum of the HRV signal sent from the heart to the brain and shifts us from the "fight or flight" mode to a calmer, more clear-minded state that facilitates social interaction. The details of this response and an explanation of the HRV frequency spectrum and why it is important will be described in detail in Chapter 4. For now, a short description of HRV is given in Box 1.1.

Based partly on the fact that the ventral vagus is neuroanatomically linked to the cranial nerves that promote social engagement, it has been hypothesized by Stephen Porges (2003) that this part of the ANS has evolved to facilitate social engagement in humans. His hypothesis, termed the polyvagal theory, together with evidence for neuroanatomical linkage of the vagus and certain other cranial nerves will be discussed later in this chapter. A diagram depicting the arrangement of all 12 cranial nerves as they leave the brain is shown in Figure 1.2.

BOX 1.1 HEART RATE VARIABILITY: DEFINITION AND IMPORTANCE

Heart rate variability (HRV) is defined as the variation in the time interval between heartbeats. Heart rate (HR) varies because sometimes the input of the sympathetic ANS nerves to the heart outweighs that of the parasympathetic branch, in which case HR increases, and sometimes the opposite happens, and HR decreases. The dynamic interplay of these two branches allows the heart to respond efficiently to different triggers and situations.

If an event stimulates your "fight or flight response," a strong sympathetic activation increases your HR and blood circulation, providing you with extra energy. During the stressful event, and for a short while afterwards, your HR settles at that higher level and parasympathetic input is insufficient to bring it down. When the ANS is functioning optimally, soon after the stress is over, the parasympathetic mode can take over, and HR decreases. However, the goal is not to remain in a parasympathetic state no matter what, because the sympathetic response should be quickly activated again when needed – for example, having to climb a flight of stairs.

If the body can quickly adapt its HR depending on the situation, that means HRV is high and your vagus nerve coordinates with your sympathetic nerves minute by minute to ensure that your blood circulation meets your needs. The continual shift from sympathetic to parasympathetic dominance causes the HR to oscillate at various frequencies, hence the term "HRV frequency spectrum." Chronic stress can impair the ongoing "conversation" between sympathetic and parasympathetic nerves, so that one component, usually the sympathetic, predominates. That means that the HR does not change much, HRV is low and the frequency spectrum is altered. Low HRV is a marker of stress.

The types of therapies that can be used to stimulate the cranial nerves, other than the vagus and its branches, are shown in Table 1.3. The olfactory nerve governs smell. The trigeminal nerve enables sensation and motor function of the face and mouth, and the facial nerve is associated with movement of the face muscles and with salivation. Both nerves will be activated by laughter yoga and by somatic therapy because somatic therapy involves talking. The auricular nerve branches off from the facial nerve and carries sensory information to the skin overlying the ear. This nerve can be accessed and stimulated by acupuncture in the ear area. The spinal accessory nerve innervates two muscles, the sternocleidomastoid and the trapezius, and controls the movement of certain neck muscles, and can be stimulated during massage. The hypoglossal nerve controls tongue muscles that help with speech and swallowing, and so this nerve is stimulated by laughter yoga, somatic therapy and social engagement.

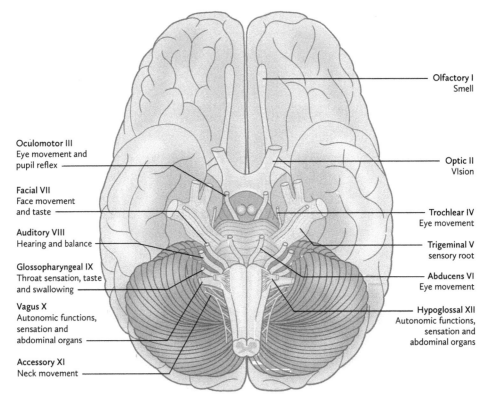

FIGURE 1.2 ARRANGEMENT OF ALL 12 CRANIAL NERVES AS THEY LEAVE THE BRAIN.
Source: Adapted from Patrick J. Lynch, medical illustrator, derivative work. Beao derivative work: Dwstultz (CC BY 2.5), via Wikimedia Commons.

Table 1.3 Therapies that stimulate each cranial nerve

Cranial nerve	Laughter yoga	Breath-work	Somatic therapy	Acu-puncture	Aroma-therapy	Massage
I Olfactory		✓			✓	
V Trigeminal	✓		✓			

Cranial nerve	Laughter yoga	Breath-work	Somatic therapy	Acu-puncture	Aroma-therapy	Massage
VII Facial	✓		✓			
VII Facial – auricular branch				✓		
XI Spinal accessory						✓
XII Hypoglossal	✓		✓			

CONNECTIONS BETWEEN THE VAGUS NERVE AND THE LIMBIC SYSTEM

The vagus nerve connects to the medulla oblongata part of the brain stem which is closely linked to the limbic system. Important structures of the limbic system can be seen in Figure 1.3, such as the hippocampus, amygdala and hypothalamus. The hippocampus is very important in the storage of memories to do with learning and remembering facts and events – declarative memory – whereas the amygdala is responsible for storing memories connected with emotion. If a memory has both a factual and an emotional content, it is much more likely to leave a deep impression than if there is no emotion attached. For example, the chances that you remember what you ate for lunch last Tuesday would be much higher if the lunch were hosted by a dear friend whom you had not seen for a while, than if you ate alone. The gratitude and appreciation you felt would add intensity to the memory and allow a more detailed recollection of the events, including the taste and texture of the moist salmon in the salad you were served. As you recall that pleasurable moment, your prefrontal cortex, or thinking part of the brain, sends that information to another part of the limbic system, the hypothalamus. This structure controls many critical bodily functions and stimulates or quietens the ANS and adrenal glands in response to signals from the prefrontal cortex.

One other part of the limbic system not shown in Figure 1.3 is the thalamus which means "inner room" in Greek. The thalamus sits on top of the brain stem and acts as a gateway to the conscious brain because nearly all sensory inputs from other areas of the nervous system – for example, from the vagus nerve – pass through it to the cerebral cortex. In this way, the limbic system connects the body to the mind and vice versa. We know that the vagus nerve engages with the limbic system, because when the vagus nerve is stimulated, the activity of the limbic system diminishes, indicating a state of low ANS arousal (Wittbrodt *et al.* 2020).

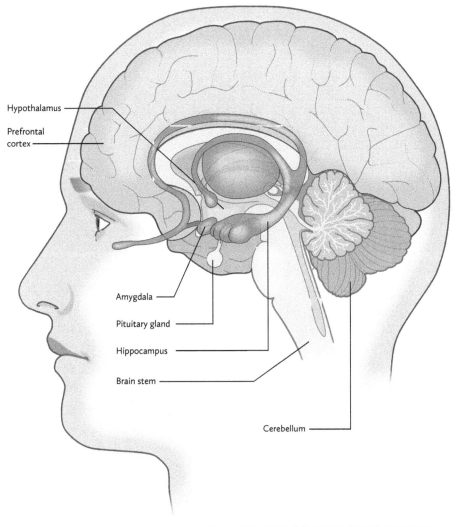

Hypothalamus

Prefrontal
cortex

Amygdala

Pituitary gland

Hippocampus

Brain stem

Cerebellum

FIGURE 1.3 SOME IMPORTANT STRUCTURES OF THE LIMBIC SYSTEM.

UNIQUENESS OF THE VAGUS NERVE

Most nerves are either motor nerves that send secretory or contraction/relaxation instructions from the brain to the target organ or tissue or sensory nerves that record information about the chemical processes and/or physical stresses occurring in the organ or tissue and transmit that information to the brain. The vagus nerve is unique because it contains *both* types of nerve fibers, motor and sensory. It is a two-way highway linking the mind and the body that enables "top-down" and "bottom-up" interactions.

In "top-down" interactions, thoughts and imagery are filtered through memory, learning and emotional areas of the limbic system. The filtered information is then received by the hypothalamus which activates the ANS and hormonal pathways and influences the biochemical responses of organ and tissue cells. For example, you may be sitting in a dentist's chair while the dentist prepares the local anesthetic she will inject into your inner mouth and gums. You remember last time you had an oral injection you felt a strange, unpleasant sensation spreading throughout your cheek, and you think that this time it will be just as bad, if not worse. Your ANS shifts to "fight or flight," and sympathetic nerves and adrenal glands are on full alert. That is a "top-down" interaction. What has that got to do with the vagus nerve? In this case, the vagal input is minimal because the vagal motor fibers are not doing very much. It is the sympathetic nervous system that is in charge.

In "bottom-up" interactions, the organs and tissues send sensory information to the brain. In this case, as you sit in the dentist's chair, you become aware that your heart is racing and you are breathing rapidly. Once again, that information is being transmitted largely through sympathetic sensory nerves, rather than through the vagal sensory fibers. Then you feel the needle enter your gum tissue and the anesthetic spreads within your oral cavity. Suddenly, you remember from reading self-help articles that distracting your mind from the present situation would probably help, so you decide to gaze at the painting of the beautiful flowers on the ceiling and appreciate the colors to take your mind off the situation. This is another "top-down" interaction, but now it is mediated through the motor *vagal* nerve fibers instead of the sympathetic "fight or flight" nerves. As a result, your heart rate and respiration rate slow down and you feel more relaxed. You have now experienced a "top-down" interaction conducted by motor fibers in the vagus nerve calming you down.

The vagus nerve is also unique in that it contains two types of motor fibers, *dorsal* and *ventral*. Dorsal fibers are unmyelinated, meaning that they are not insulated by a fatty, myelin sheath and they carry out slow but smooth conduction of nerve impulses. Generally, they foster digestion after each meal, but they also respond to threat or novel situations by reducing cardiac output to save metabolic resources. This latter reaction is associated with immobilization behaviors and is termed the "freeze response." It occurs when something is so frightening that our brains decide we cannot take on the threat, nor are we able to escape. As a result, our bodies remain still, unable to move, and sometimes we cannot speak. On the other hand, ventral fibers are myelinated and can transmit information faster, allowing for the occurrence of more complex brain processes.

Ventral nerve fibers in the inferior cardiac vagal nerve rapidly regulate cardiac output, by periodically sending parasympathetic inputs to the heart, momentarily slowing heart rate and reducing contractility. In this way, the ventral vagus acts as a brake in which rapid engagement and disengagement of vagal stimulus to the heart can quickly mobilize or calm an individual. This allows the person to rapidly engage or disengage with objects and other people and to promote self-soothing behaviors. The resulting natural interplay between the sympathetic and parasympathetic systems allows the heart to quickly adapt to different situations and needs, and HRV is increased, as will be described in more detail in Chapter 4.

BASIC FUNCTIONS OF THE DIFFERENT FIBERS

The cranial nerves, including the vagus, are attached to the brain stem through aggregates of cells called brain stem nuclei located in the medulla oblongata part of the brain stem. These nuclei aid in the transfer of motor and sensory information between body organs and structures and the limbic system. As described above, nerve fibers can be motor (sometimes known as *afferent* – meaning signaling from the brain to the organ) or sensory (sometimes known as *efferent* – meaning signaling from the organ to the brain). Cranial nerves can be either motor or sensory, or can be mixed, as in the vagus nerve. Cranial nerves with motor (efferent) functions are grouped according to the structures they innervate as follows:

- general somatic efferents (GSE)
- special visceral efferents (SVE)
- general visceral efferents (GVE).

General somatic efferent fibers signal to our skin and skeletal muscles, including those in our face and tongue, while *general visceral* efferent fibers signal mainly to our internal organs, specifically to the smooth muscle cells of airways and blood vessels, to cardiac muscle and to secretory glands such as those in the intestine and endocrine system. *Special visceral* efferent nerves are an exception regarding target organs because they innervate the striated muscles of the head and neck (branchial) rather than the internal organs. There are no special somatic efferent nerve fibers.

Similarly, cranial nerves with sensory (afferent) functions are grouped according to the structures from which they receive information as follows:

- general somatic afferents (GSA)
- special somatic afferents (SSA)
- general visceral afferents (GVA)
- special visceral afferents (SVA).

If a nerve fiber exclusively carries sensory information from our special senses (vision, smell, taste, hearing and balance), it is called a *special somatic afferent nerve*. If it carries other types of sensory information, like touch, pressure, pain, temperature, then it is a *general somatic afferent nerve*. General somatic afferent nerve fibers convey impulses to the brain associated with the cutaneous sensations of pain, temperature, touch, vibration or pressure and from proprioceptors localized in the muscles, joints and ligaments. Special somatic afferent fibers carry sensory information from the special senses of vision, hearing and balance. *General visceral afferent* fibers convey visceral information such as distention of organs and chemical conditions from the blood vessels, heart, lungs, digestive system and other organ systems and glands. *Special visceral afferents* develop in association with the intestine and carry the special senses of smell and taste.

The brain stem nuclei to which nerve fibers are connected depend on whether the fibers are motor or sensory; ventral motor or dorsal motor; somatic or visceral; or special or general. In the brain stem, there are about 18 cranial nerve nuclei comprising ten motor cranial nerve nuclei and eight sensory cranial nerve nuclei. Table 1.4 describes the brain stem nuclei that are important for self-regulation and the functions that they regulate.

Table 1.4 Brain stem nuclei and how they relate to self-regulation

Brain stem nucleus	Type of nerve fiber	Function
Motor nucleus of facial nerve	General somatic efferent	Facial movement and expression, salivation
Motor nucleus of trigeminal nerve	Special visceral efferent	Chewing and swallowing, facial expression
Motor nucleus of glossopharyngeal nerve	Special visceral efferent	Phonation (voice), salivation
Dorsal motor nucleus	General visceral efferent (dorsal)	Involuntary muscle control (intestinal muscle – peristalsis; airway muscles – respiration; cardiac muscle – dorsal freeze response) Secretory gland control (i.e., digestion)

Brain stem nucleus	Type of nerve fiber	Function
Nucleus ambiguus	General and special visceral efferent (ventral)	Cardiovascular regulation, phonation
Nucleus tractus solitarius	Special visceral afferent	Taste and smell (olfaction)
Nucleus tractus solitarius	General visceral afferent	Visceral sensibility (heart and intestine)
Nucleus spinal tract V	General somatic afferent	Cutaneous sensibility

To summarize Table 1.4, the dorsal motor nucleus supplies parasympathetic efferents primarily to the gastrointestinal tract and lungs, although dorsal nerve fibers are in place in the cardiac branches to enable the freeze response (sharp reduction in cardiac output and metabolic expenditure) in the case of severe psychological stress. The ventral efferent fibers that arise from the nucleus ambiguus supply preganglionic parasympathetic neurons to the heart which when stimulated produce a periodic parasympathetic input that increases HRV, leading to improved cardiac function, mental acuity and emotional regulation. This is a key pathway by which many techniques for self-regulation, such as mindfulness and gratitude, are mediated.

The nucleus ambiguus is a composite nucleus that also contributes fibers to the glossopharyngeal and accessory nerves serving the muscles of the soft palate, pharynx, larynx and neck. This means that the same ventral vagal soothing mechanisms that are set in motion in the heart can also be accessed by voice (laughter yoga, chanting, somatic therapy), respiration (breath control) and neck movement (massage, yoga, somatic therapy). The nucleus solitarius receives primary afferents from visceral organs, as well as information about taste and smell, and so plays a major role in manifesting the influences of aromatherapy as well as colon hydrotherapy and modulation of diet on mood. The nucleus spinal tract V receives information on cutaneous sensibility and is instrumental in mediating the effects of acupuncture on the skin overlying the ear on pain relief and calming the mind.

THE POLYVAGAL THEORY

The polyvagal theory was introduced by behavioral neuroscientist, Stephen W. Porges, in his presidential address to the Society of Psychophysiological Research in Atlanta, Georgia on October 8, 1994. It is based on three evolutionary stages of the ANS:

1. A primitive unmyelinated visceral vagus that fosters digestion and responds to threat by depressing metabolic activity (dorsal vagus).
2. A sympathetic nervous system that is capable of increasing metabolic output and inhibiting the visceral vagus to foster mobilization behaviors necessary for "fight or flight."
3. A myelinated vagus that *can rapidly regulate cardiac output* to foster engagement and disengagement with the environment. This vagus is neuroanatomically linked to the cranial nerves that regulate social engagement via facial expression and vocalization (ventral vagal complex).

An important point is that the polyvagal theory emphasizes the neurophysiological and neuroanatomical distinction between two branches of the vagus, dorsal and ventral, and proposes that each branch supports different types of behavioral strategies to cope with stress. The social engagement system (ventral vagal complex) puts the brakes on the other (fight, flight, freeze) strategies, thus keeping our heart and body active while we work through a situation. On the other hand, the social engagement system will release the brakes to engage a different response to the environment (i.e., running) if engagement doesn't help to get us into a safe situation. The three evolutionary stages of the ANS are summarized in Figure 1.4 in terms of a tiered response to threat, with the most primitive phase at the bottom.

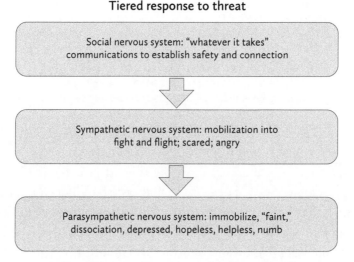

Tiered response to threat

Social nervous system: "whatever it takes" communications to establish safety and connection

Sympathetic nervous system: mobilization into fight and flight; scared; angry

Parasympathetic nervous system: immobilize, "faint," dissociation, depressed, hopeless, helpless, numb

FIGURE 1.4 TIERED RESPONSE TO THREAT.
Source: Adapted from Schwartz A, 2020. Polyvagal theory in psychotherapy: practical applications for PTSD treatment. https://drarielleschwartz.com/ polyvagal-theory-in-psychotherapy-dr-arielle-schwartz/#.Yp6AKxPMJ_Q.

The parasympathetic system is the oldest stage, reflecting the survival needs of a primitive passive feeder. Stress responses are primarily limited to adjusting the metabolic rate within a fairly narrow range, and "death feigning" survival tactics. The sympathetic nervous system is a later development, adding mobility, mobilization and a wider range of possible survival responses. This system shifts resources to muscular, visceral or other systems as needed in response to survival challenges. The most recent stage, the "social nervous system," developed *in mammals only,* regulates the sympathetic system and moderates the "fight or flight" responses enabling social interactions between newborn and mother and, later, social cooperation and engagement between people in general. These three stages differ both in the degree of ANS arousal – high energy or low energy – and the perceived emotional valence – a feeling of safety and security or of threat – as illustrated in Figure 1.5.

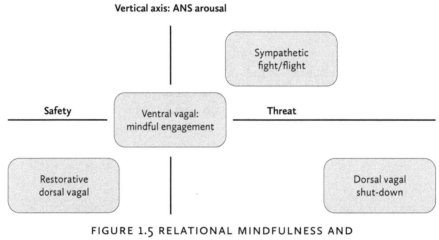

FIGURE 1.5 RELATIONAL MINDFULNESS AND
THE AUTONOMIC NERVOUS SYSTEM.
*Source: Relational Mindfulness & The Autonomic Nervous
System (ANS) © 2018 ProactiveMindfulness.com.*

Dorsal shut-down, or freeze response, is low in energy and high in threat. The immobilization, loss of muscle tone, slowed heart rate, nausea, dizziness and numbness resemble "feigned death" and may even be a lifesaver in the case of a person who is in the presence of an intruder who wants them dead. Sympathetic "fight or flight" is associated with a moderate degree of threat and the energy level is raised to enable a rapid escape. Ventral vagal mindful engagement is the balanced state right in the middle of sympathetic and parasympathetic stimulation, a state of "relaxed alertness" where you are ready for anything. This condition is similar to the readiness of a good tennis player who positions themselves close to the net, right in the center, so they can reach for the ball from whichever direction it approaches them.

A fourth state is shown here – "restorative dorsal vagal" – which is not a response to threat but a resting low-energy mode that is achieved in safe situations and is essential for long-term mind-body repair and maintenance. Basically, "ventral vagal" is the optimum state for day-to-day functioning, with "fight or flight" being a necessary higher-energy level for dealing with emergencies and meeting deadlines. Problems arise when "fight or flight" becomes the usual "go-to" state. The ventral vagal state can be subdivided into varying degrees of arousal and valence all within an acceptable degree of ANS balance, as shown in Figure 1.6.

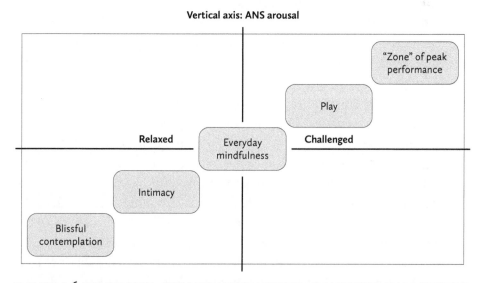

FIGURE 1.6 RELATIONAL MINDFULNESS: STATES OF MINDFUL ENGAGEMENT.
Source: Relational Mindfulness: States of Mindful Engagement © 2018 ProactiveMindfulness.com.

In Figure 1.6, the horizontal axis has been changed to "relaxed" and "challenged" rather than "safety" and "threat." Everyday mindfulness is right in the middle, between relaxed and challenged, and is associated with a moderate degree of energy. This is the perfect state for enjoying your day, maintaining good health and successfully dealing with minor problems. Ideally, a little more challenge is met with a corresponding increase in energy level, such as needed to progress from a friendly game of tennis to competing in a series to get to the next level. On the other end of the scale, a little more relaxation opens one up to enhanced social interaction. You no longer rush past the man who sells newspapers on the corner, but you take the time to look him in the eyes, smile and wish him a good day. Choosing to relax even further, perhaps in a meditation class, you expend even less energy and may open up to non-verbal communication with those around you.

The key new concept that Porges introduced in the polyvagal theory is that a myelinated vagus *rapidly regulates cardiac output* to foster engagement and disengagement with the environment. This means that the heart is no longer just a pump that continually supplies the body with blood containing adequate oxygen, glucose, nutrients and hormones. At first sight, it may seem that conscious thoughts in the brain initiate the choice to foster engagement and disengagement with the environment. However, if you are experiencing the "fight or flight" response, your heart is in sympathetic overdrive, your HRV is low, and this information is sent from the heart to the brain via the sympathetic nervous system to put the brain on alert. This is no time to engage with the environment other than to check to make sure that you have an escape route, either in the real world or metaphorically. Your world view is narrowed down and focused purely on getting yourself out of trouble. (Heart-to-brain communication and how it alters brain function is explored more fully in Chapter 4.)

In order for a person to be physiologically equipped for genuine engagement with the environment, the heart needs to receive periodic input from the vagus nerve so that the sympathetic and parasympathetic systems are in constant communication, allowing the heart to adapt to the needs of the mind and the body on a second-by-second basis. The presence of this communication is reflected in the frequency spectrum of the HRV signal that is sent from the heart to the brain through the sympathetic spinal afferents and the vagus nerve. As described in Chapter 4, when this signal reaches the thalamus, it optimizes the ability to focus on the present moment and improves cognitive skills and memory recall, all of which enhance the ability to engage with the environment and socially interact.

Another concept that Porges introduces in the polyvagal theory is that the ventral vagus nerve is neuroanatomically linked to the cranial nerves that regulate social engagement via facial expression and vocalization. In support of this statement, recent research confirms that the nucleus ambiguus is the common nucleus of the efferent fibers from the glossopharyngeal and vagus nerves (Petko and Tadi 2022). The glossopharyngeal nerve regulates salivation and use of voice, both of which are employed during social interactions that include eating. In addition, the spinal trigeminal nucleus that receives its main input from the trigeminal nerve also has an additional connection to the vagus nerve (Baker and Lui 2022). The linkage of the glossopharyngeal and trigeminal nerves to the ventral vagus fibers means that the processes of chewing, swallowing, speaking and making facial expressions, which are all associated with social interaction, are stimulated at the same time that the heart is being calmed and prepared for engagement by input from the ventral vagus nerve fibers.

Although the polyvagal theory makes sense regarding mind-body interactions, it is still a theory rather than proven fact. The traditional view of the ANS is based on a two-part system: the sympathetic nervous system, which is more activating and enables the "fight or flight" response, and the parasympathetic nervous system, the main nerve being the vagus nerve, which supports digestion and repair ("rest and digest"). No mention is made of a "social engagement system" in which ventral fibers in the vagus nerve rhythmically relax the heart to promote a state of "relaxed alertness" conducive to engagement, and coordinate with cranial nerves that foster social behaviors. In addition, more focus is on the motor components of the ANS, minimizing the important role of afferent and limbic contributions to the regulation of the body's organs and tissues. This bias neglects the feedback system in which the visceral and other organs inform the limbic system and cortex of the brain about their local physical and chemical environment, which is necessary for maintenance of homeostasis.

However, critics of the polyvagal theory indicate that its principles are not supported by empirical, scientific research. Paul Grossman of University Hospital Basel, argues that there is no evidence that the dorsal motor nucleus is an evolutionarily more primitive center of the brain stem parasympathetic system than the nucleus ambiguus, and that no evidence supports the claim that a sudden decrease in heart rate elicited by extreme stress is due to dorsal vagal fiber efferent activity to the heart (Grossman and Taylor 2007). Other investigators argue that "a differentiation of the visceral efferent column of the vagus nerve into a dorsal motor nucleus and a ventrolateral nucleus (nucleus ambiguus) was first seen in reptiles" (Barbas-Henry and Lohman 1984).

These criticisms undermine the idea that there is a phylogenetic hierarchy, in which one vagal system is more primitive than the other and therefore is activated only when the more evolved one fails. They also contradict the claim that the nucleus ambiguus is unique to mammals. These critics argue that the proposed anatomical difference between the vagus nerve origins of mammals versus other vertebrates would be an insufficient basis for explaining complex social and emotional behavior differences observed.

Even among critics, there seems to be little if any disagreement with the key concepts proposed by Porges:

- A myelinated vagus *rapidly regulates cardiac output* to "foster engagement and disengagement with the environment."
- The ventral vagus nerve is "neuroanatomically linked to the cranial nerves that regulate social engagement via facial expression and vocalization."

Nor is there much argument with the idea, based on the above concepts, that a "social nervous system" regulates the sympathetic system and moderates the "fight or flight" responses enabling social interactions between newborn and mother and, later, social cooperation and engagement between people in general. This is the most important and useful part of the polyvagal theory, regardless of whether one part of the vagal system is more primitive than the other. In summary, the polyvagal theory is not an established fact and needs to be further developed and amended according to future relevant research findings. However, it does provide a useful perspective from which to interpret HRV and to develop therapies to optimize day-to-day functioning in a challenging world.

REFERENCES

Baker E and Lui F, 2022. Neuroanatomy, vagal nerve nuclei. In: StatPearls [Internet]. Treasure Island (FL): StatPearls Publishing. Available from: www.ncbi.nlm.nih.gov/books/NBK545209.

Barbas-Henry H and Lohman AH, 1984. The motor nuclei and primary projections of the IXth, Xth, XIth, and XIIth cranial nerves in the monitor lizard, Varanus exanthematicus. *Journal of Comparative Neurology.* 226(4): 565–579. doi: 10.1002/cne.902260409.

Grossman P and Taylor EW, 2007. Toward understanding respiratory sinus arrhyhmia: relations to cardiac vagal tone, evolution and biobehavioral functions. *Biological Psychology.* 74(2): 263–285. doi: 10.1016/j.biopsycho.2005.11.014.

Petko B and Tadi P, 2022. Neuroanatomy, nucleus ambiguus. In: StatPearls [Internet]. Treasure Island (FL): StatPearls Publishing. Available from: https://pubmed.ncbi.nlm.nih.gov/31613524.

Porges SW, 2003. Social engagement and attachment. A phylogenetic perspective. *Ann N Y Acad Sci.* 1008: 31–47. doi: 10.1196/annals.1301.004.

Wittbrodt MT, Gurel NZ, Nye JA *et al.*, 2020. Non-invasive vagal nerve stimulation decreases brain activity during trauma scripts. *Brain Stimulation.* 13(5): P1333–1348. doi: 10.1016/j. brs.2020.07.002.

CHAPTER 2

Cranial Branches

ACUPUNCTURE, AROMATHERAPY AND MASSAGE

In this chapter, we will focus on three of the cranial nerves: the facial (VII), the olfactory (I) and the spinal accessory (XI) nerves. We are specifically interested in the anterior auricular branch of the facial nerve that provides sensory information to the skin overlying the ear. This nerve can be stimulated by applying an acupuncture needle in the inferior concha, or shell-shaped structure, of the cavity of the external ear. When this nerve is activated, it sends sensory information to small nerves in the nucleus solitarius connected to the brain stem. These small nerves connect with vagal efferent nerves in the nucleus ambiguus and the dorsal motor nucleus that propagate the vagal stimulus to the sinoatrial node of the heart. As a result, heart rate decreases as part of the "rest and digest" parasympathetic response.

The olfactory nerve is also of interest because it can be stimulated by aromatherapy. Each aroma has a specific effect on this nerve and on the olfactory bulb. For example, lavender usually promotes a calm, peaceful attitude, whereas peppermint prevents fatigue. Interestingly, the olfactory nerve is also linked to the nucleus solitarius that receives sensory information from the intestine. It has been suggested that olfactory and visceral functions interact in the nucleus tractus solitarius, modulating taste mechanisms involved in food selection and ingestion (Garcia-Diaz *et al.* 1988). This means that smelling a particular aroma – for example, cinnamon – may trigger the same sensory signal from your intestinal nerves to your brain as if you had eaten a cinnamon roll, adding to the pleasurable sensation you experience if you like the smell of cinnamon.

The spinal accessory innervates the sternocleidomastoid muscles on each side of the neck as well as the trapezius muscles on top of the shoulders. The former muscles help to rotate the head and keep it aligned with the spine, and the latter control movement of the head, neck and shoulders. Both sets of muscles can be manipulated by massage, and as a result the spinal accessory nerve is activated. Since the spinal accessory nerve appears to have fibers connecting to the vagus nerve, this may be the reason that massage of the head, neck and shoulders increases vagal tone and reduces heart rate, as will be demonstrated later in this chapter.

AURICULAR STIMULATION WITH ACUPUNCTURE

Popularity of acupuncture

According to Oxford Languages, acupuncture is "a system of complementary medicine in which fine needles are inserted in the skin at specific points along what are considered to be lines of energy (meridians), used in the treatment of various physical and mental conditions." Although the practice of acupuncture evolved in ancient China, during the last 40 to 50 years acupuncture has become more and more popular in the West. In 2021, the National Institute of Health and Clinical Excellence (NICE) recommended acupuncture as an option for treatment of chronic pain in the UK (NICE 2021).

According to the National Health Service, acupuncture is used in many NHS general practitioner practices, as well as in most pain clinics and hospices in the UK. In the USA, the number of acupuncture users and licensed acupuncturists increased by 50 percent and 100 percent respectively between 2002 and 2012, coinciding with increasing acknowledgement of the importance and efficacy of acupuncture over this period (Cui *et al.* 2017). There has been a steady linear increase in acupuncture usage from 2002 to 2012, which continues to the present day (Miller *et al.* 2021). Its rise in popularity, particularly in the West, is partly due to its effectiveness for pain relief in real-world conditions and partly because scientific studies have begun to show its efficacy in ideal, controlled conditions.

History of acupuncture

An excellent summary of the history of acupuncture can be found in Hao and Mittleman's paper "Acupuncture Past, Present and Future" (2014). Briefly, the ancient practice of acupuncture started in China approximately 3000 years ago (Kirchhof-Glazier n.d.). A drawing from a Chinese manuscript in the Bibliothèque Nationale de France indicates acupuncture points (Figure 2.1).

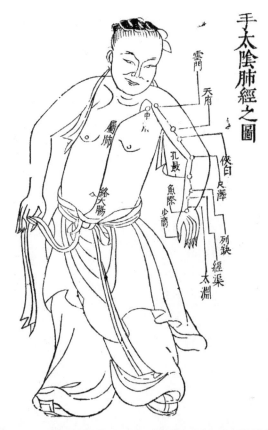

FIGURE 2.1 DRAWING FROM A CHINESE MANUSCRIPT
SHOWING ACUPUNCTURE POINTS.
Source: Courtesy of the Bibliothèque Nationale de France, Paris. https://cdn.britannica.com/45/77345-050-A66D0717/Acupuncture-points-manuscript-Chinese-Bibliotheque-Nationale-de.jpg.

Acupuncture was first documented in *The Yellow Emperor's Classic of Internal Medicine*, by Huangdi Neijing in 100 BCE in which it was described as an organized system of diagnosis and treatment. By this time, the idea of Qi (vital energy or life force) flow channels in the body was well established, and the principles of acupuncture probably evolved from the addition of a collection of traditions passed down over centuries (Baldry 1993). Gradually, the practice of acupuncture was perfected until it became a standard practice in China along with massage, dietary manipulation and herbs. In the sixth century CE, acupuncture spread to Korea and then to Japan, but it took a while to reach the West.

The first medical description of acupuncture by a European was in about 1680 by a Dutch doctor, Willem ten Rhijne, who worked for the East India Company and witnessed acupuncture practice in Japan (White and Ernst 2004; Bivens 2000). The result was his book *Dissertatio de Arthritide*, published in London in

1683, which included a very important treatise on acupuncture (Figure 2.2). He portrayed Japanese practitioners with a sense of awe because they were able to use this therapy to treat the same diseases that were treated in Europe by the detested practice of bloodletting.

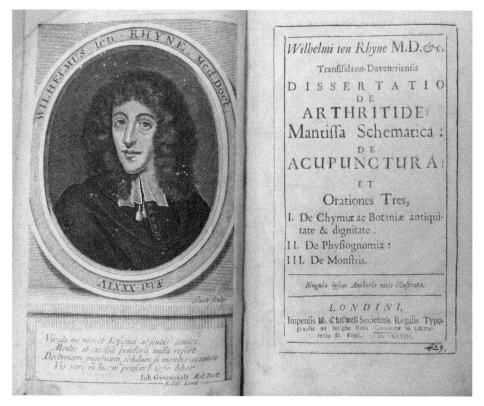

FIGURE 2.2 *DISSERTATIO DE ARTHRITIDE* BY
WILLEM TEN RHIJNE, LONDON, 1683.
Source: Courtesy of Rare Books Collection, Falk Library of the Health Sciences, University of Pittsburgh. https://info.hsls.pitt.edu/updatereport/files/2015/01/Rhijne1.jpg.

For nearly 300 years after this publication, interest in acupuncture was minimal in the United States, until it was used on a US Press Corps member after he received an emergency appendectomy in Beijing, China (Reston 1971). Following this, teams of US physicians toured China to learn more about acupuncture and its benefits, especially regarding its use for surgical analgesia (Dimond 1971). When it proved at the time to be unreliable, enthusiasm waned, and acupuncture was deemed to be a sham practice. Despite this, patients for whom conventional treatments were ineffective turned to acupuncture hoping that it might offer relief.

Gradually, more and more patients experienced positive effects from acupuncture, and studies were conducted proving its efficacy in pain management and in relief of nausea, and a National Institutes of Health consensus conference reported positive evidence for the effectiveness of acupuncture (NIH 1997). In a recent thorough review of acupuncture research, the NIH and NICE concluded that clinical evidence showed a benefit of acupuncture compared to both sham acupuncture and usual care in reducing pain and improving quality of life (NICE 2020).

Anatomy of the ear

The external ear is the location in the body where the vagus nerve sends its only peripheral branch. Stemming from this branch is an array of vagal afferent (sensory) nerves within the skin that provides an ideal route for non-invasive vagal nerve stimulation. Currently, the literature lacks a clear agreement on the auricular sites that are most densely innervated by these nerves, and that is a disadvantage, but it is generally thought that the concha and inner tragus are suitable locations for vagal stimulation. Figure 2.3 shows the locations of these structures (left) and the areas served by different auricular nerves (right).

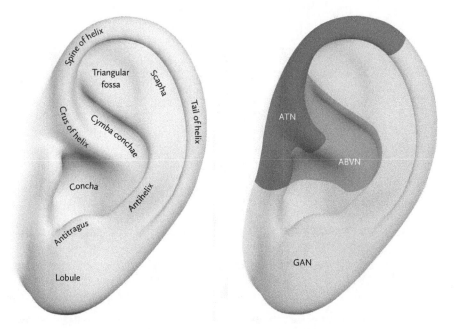

FIGURE 2.3 ANATOMY OF THE EAR AND ITS NERVES.
ATN, auriculotemporal nerve; ABVN, auricular branch vagal nerve; GAN, great auricular nerve.
Source: Adapted from Butt et al. 2020, Figure 1.

Auricular acupuncture for vagal stimulation

Ear acupuncture is performed using fine, sterilized needles of varying lengths which are inserted into specific acupoints of the auricle. According to the UK Health Centre (n.d.), these needles can be left in for anywhere between 30–40 minutes and a few days; however, most treatments last less than one hour. If the objective is just to stimulate the vagus nerve, only one or two needles are usually employed. This treatment is regularly reviewed for safety and has not presented any major concerns in the UK so far. Provided that the acupuncturist follows their training and uses sterile needles in a hygienic environment, the risk of infection after auricular acupuncture is extremely small.

Evidence that auricular acupuncture increases vagal tone

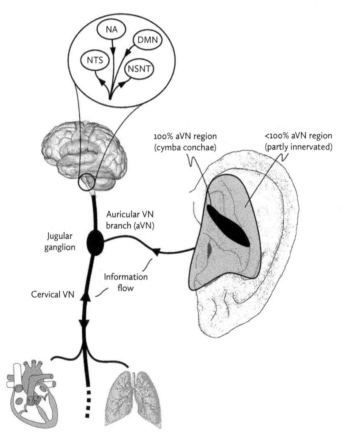

FIGURE 2.4 CONNECTION OF THE EAR TO THE VAGUS NERVE.
NA, nucleus ambiguus; NTS, nucleus tractus solitarius; DMN, dorsal motor nucleus; NSNT, nucleus spinalis of the trigeminal nerve; VN, vagal nerve; aVN, afferent auricular branches.
Source: Kaniusas et al. 2019, Figure 1A. CC BY 4.0.

The exact way in which auricular acupuncture increases vagal tone has not been defined, but two possible mechanisms have been proposed that are consistent with the anatomy and physiology of the ear and its connections to the ANS. In one case, acupuncture causes the auricular nerve branch to send sensory information to the main vagus nerve, and vagal afferent nerves transmit that information to the nucleus tractus solitarius (NTS). This signal stimulates efferent nerves in the dorsal vagal nucleus (DVN) and nucleus ambiguus (NA) to propagate vagal tone to the sinoatrial node of the heart resulting in decreased heart rate and enhanced HRV. A diagram to illustrate this process is shown in Figure 2.4.

In addition, the nucleus solitarius neurons may activate the caudal ventro-lateral medulla (CVLM) and consequently inhibit the rostroventrolateral medulla (RVLM) that is responsible for exciting the sympathetic preganglionic nerves in the spinal column (Figure 2.5). In this way, sympathetic activity decreases, also reducing heart rate and enhancing HRV.

The alternative proposed mechanism is that auricular acupuncture directly stimulates vagal efferent nerves from the ear which then activate the vagus nerve so that it increases parasympathetic input to the heart, slowing down heart rate and increasing HRV.

The effectiveness of auricular acupuncture on improving vagal tone is often calibrated using HRV because there is a direct correlation between the magnitude of HRV, measured as the standard deviation of inter-beat intervals (SDNN) and vagal tone. Another HRV parameter that reflects vagal tone is how quickly heart rate varies on a beat-to-beat basis, known as RMSSD (root mean square of successive differences between inter-beat intervals). This is because the vagal response is mediated by release of the neurotransmitter acetylcholine (ACH), which acts very quickly compared to the sympathetic neurotransmitter, norepinephrine. The effect of ACH on the heart is felt within the period of a single heartbeat, unlike the effect of norepinephrine which is mediated over 5–15 seconds. Therefore, if there are large differences in successive inter-beat intervals, RMSSD will be high, reflecting increased release of ACH leading to high vagal tone. On the same basis, the degree of vagal tone is reflected in the frequency domain of HRV. Since acetylcholine is a fast-acting neurotransmitter, it changes heart rate on a beat-to-beat basis causing high frequency (HF) changes in HRV.

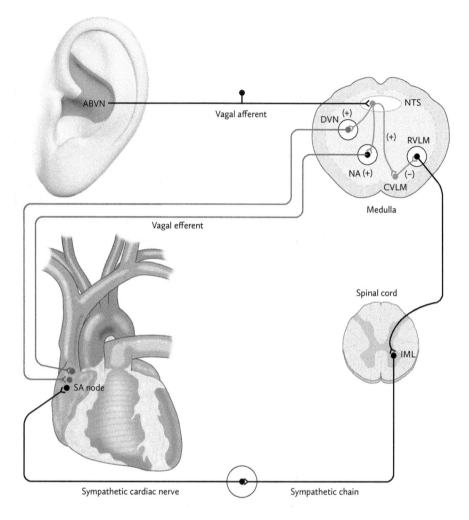

FIGURE 2.5 NEURAL CONNECTION OF THE EAR TO THE HEART.
Source: Adapted from Butt et al. 2020, Figure 6.

Based on its effects on HRV, there is some evidence that auricular acupuncture increases vagal tone. One study was performed on 24 healthy men who received auricular acupuncture for 30 minutes in which a needle was applied to the inferior concha of the ear. They also received placebo acupuncture at the Ma35 point which is used to treat pain caused by gonarthrosis, or cartilage damage to the knee joint (Boehmer *et al.* 2020). Half of the participants received placebo acupuncture two days before the auricular acupuncture, and the others two days afterwards. HRV was measured during, and immediately after, both procedures. Measurement of HRV without acupuncture (no-treatment control) was performed under the same conditions in 12 randomly selected subjects from the 24 subjects in the main analysis after completion of both acupuncture measurements. The results indicated that their parasympathetic nervous system, or vagal tone, was significantly stimulated by auricular acupuncture as shown by a marked reduction in heart rate and an increase in SDNN during and after auricular acupuncture as compared to placebo or no treatment. However, no effect was found on the frequency-domain HRV parameters, and it was concluded that the vagal effect observed in this experiment must be modest, requiring further investigation.

On the other hand, in a controlled study on 26 patients who had auricular acupuncture at the "Shenmen" and "Point Zero" points (shown in Figure 2.6) after undergoing hemicolectomy surgery, a procedure to remove one side of the colon, parasympathetic activation was indicated by a significant increase in the frequency domain HRV parameter, HF, the high frequency contribution to the frequency spectrum of HRV (Arai *et al.* 2013). In addition, the ratio of sympathetic to parasympathetic stimulation, LF/HF, was significantly reduced. It was concluded that auricular acupuncture kept the LF/HF ratio at lower levels and HF at higher levels during the postoperative period, demonstrating a shift to the "rest and digest" mode. An acupuncture-induced vagal response would especially benefit patients after surgery because it would make them feel calmer and less anxious and would facilitate cellular repair.

Based on these and earlier studies, modern clinical and basic research is confirming the efficacy of ear acupuncture in treating anxiety-related disorders, such as preoperative anxiety (Wang *et al.* 2001), insomnia (Sok and Kim 2005) and dental anxiety (Karst *et al.* 2007). A recent review of 15 studies with 1603 patients concluded that: "auricular stimulation (AS) may be useful in treatment of preoperative anxiety. Due to heterogenous certainty in effect estimates, further research is needed to clarify the actual efficacy of AS for preoperative anxiety" (Usichenko *et al.* 2022). It should be noted that in this case the term

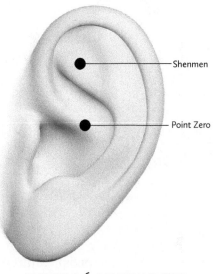

FIGURE 2.6 ACUPUNCTURE
POINTS IN THE EAR.
Source: Arai et al. 2013, Figure 1.

"auricular stimulation" includes electroacupuncture and acupressure as well as simple acupuncture.

Another review, focusing on electrical stimulation of the auricular vagus nerve (Kaniusas *et al.* 2019), ends with the following summary:

> Auricular vagus nerve stimulation is not close to prime time but gains momentum as a new way of treatment by harnessing the body's own protective mechanisms beyond the mediation of symptoms, warranting further scientific and clinical research on aVNS. aVNS makes it possible to modulate the mind's great influence over the body via the vagus nerve.

At this point, I think that auricular acupuncture may not be the most effective non-invasive complementary therapy to reduce anxiety, but it does appear to stimulate the vagus nerve and may become a useful technique in the future if more scientific evidence for efficacy is acquired.

OLFACTORY STIMULATION WITH AROMATHERAPY

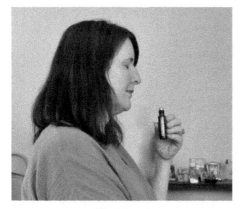

FIGURE 2.7 RECEIVING AROMPATHERAPY IN A MIND-BODY HEALTH CENTER.

Aromatherapy refers to the use of volatile ingredients from aromatic plants that have been shown to enhance physiological processes in some way in people or animals. The aromatic essences are usually simply inhaled from the container or dissolved in water and dispersed in the air using a diffuser. Sometimes they are applied topically to the skin, but care must be taken regarding correct dilution. Information about safe usage of aromatic essences is available on the website of the International Federation of Professional Aromatherapists (https://ifparoma.org). Aromatherapy is used to treat a variety of conditions in a wide range of settings, including health spas, hospitals and massage clinics (Figure 2.7).

As a rule, aromatherapy seems to relieve pain, improve mood and promote a sense of relaxation. Scientific research is showing that using aromatherapy in doctors' and dentists' waiting rooms positively affects patient satisfaction and well-being. Ambient odors of orange and lavender are much more conducive to relaxation than smells of antiseptic and cleaning supplies (Lehrner *et al.* 2005). Personally, I can vouch that waiting in a salon for a haircut is a much more pleasant and settling experience for me if I am inhaling dispersed fragrant essential oils rather than the acrid smells of hair products. In addition, it has long been known that aromatherapy can reduce the amount of time that patients perceive they have spent in the waiting room by 20 percent (Hornik 1984).

So, inhaling pure, carefully selected and appropriately diluted essential oils seems to be an easy, effortless way to make you feel relaxed and pleasantly at ease. How does this work? A possibility is that odors from plants bring us back to our place in nature. Edward O. Wilson, who was an eminent biologist, naturalist and author from Harvard University, proposed the biophilia hypothesis, which is the belief that humans are genetically predisposed to be attracted to nature. It states that all humans inherently love the natural world. How do you feel when you look at the photos of flowers in Figure 2.8?

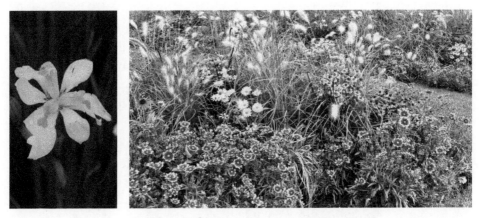

FIGURE 2.8 PHOTOS OF FLOWERS.

Maybe you feel calmer and less stressed? There is much evidence as provided by Beukeboom *et al.* (2012), and by other authors cited in their article, that just placing photographs of plants on the walls of hospital waiting rooms will significantly reduce patient anxiety. The concept of biophilia is gaining in popularity. As I am writing this chapter, I look up and see the following advertisement from the Oxford Botanic Garden & Arboretum: "An hour and a half of meditation and discovery in the Garden, using the power of plants and their essential oils to enhance your experience and connect more deeply with nature."

Perhaps because most people in Western society spend most of their time indoors and separate themselves from the living world, many are feeling a loss and are now striving to reconnect with nature through aromatherapy. According to Statista: "The market value of essential oils is expected to grow from around 17 billion U.S. dollars in 2017 to about 27 billion dollars by 2022" (Statista 2022).

Origin of aromatherapy

The use of aromatherapy for medicinal purposes started more than 6000 years ago in ancient Egypt, the Far East, China and Europe (Cerrato 1998). According to the International Federation of Aromatherapists (2023):

> The therapeutic use of aromatic plants seems to be as old as human civilization itself. Plants such as fennel, coriander seeds, cumin and many others have been found at the sites of ancient burial grounds. Many texts from Asia to Ancient Egypt, and much of the Mediterranean area, describe the various procedures and rituals involved in the making of healing ointments, medicated oils, poultices and healing perfumes.

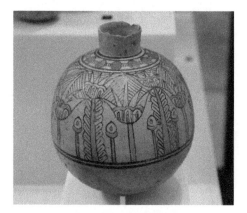

FIGURE 2.9 ANCIENT EGYPTIAN HEALING POT.
Source: Egyptian Gallery, Neues Museum, Berlin, Germany. CC0 1.0 Universal Public Domain Dedication.

The ancient Egyptians are generally regarded as the pioneers of the use of aromatic plants. They used fragrant oils in incense, medicine, massage, skincare products and cosmetics, and in their highly refined process of embalming the dead. When the tomb of Tutankhamen was opened in 1922 by Howard Carter and his team, several pots and jars were discovered that still contained scented healing salves of frankincense, Indian spikenard and kyphi, a mixture of 23 ingredients that "lulled one to sleep, allayed anxieties and brightened dreams." They had been sealed for over 3000 years. An example of an Egyptian healing pot is shown in Figure 2.9

How does aromatherapy stimulate the vagus nerve?

There are many animal and human clinical studies which show that aroma-therapy can strongly affect the ANS and that certain products reduce the "fight or flight" response by activating the parasympathetic or vagus nerve response. Part of the mechanism that enables this response is the slowing and deepening of the breath that happens when you inhale the essence. Inhaling a pleasant aroma, such as lavender, increases tidal volume, or the average volume of air inspired during a single breath, resulting in slower, deeper breathing (Masaoka *et al.* 2013). As will be explained in more detail in Chapter 4, just breathing more deeply and slowly than usual will calm your ANS by activating the vagus nerve. When stimulated, the vagus nerve releases acetylcholine which slows heart rate and alleviates anxiety. But the calming effects of aromatherapy are not just due to these changes in breathing.

From an evolutionary standpoint, olfaction is the most primal of our five senses. It is the *only sense* that connects directly with the amygdala, or the emotional processing part of the limbic system. When an essential oil aromatic vapor is inhaled, its molecules bind to the receptors in the nasal cavity. Olfactory sensory nerves then transmit the signal to the olfactory bulb that filters and processes the signal. The olfactory bulb is where olfactory nerves integrate the sensory information they are receiving from the receptors in the nasal cavity. As shown in Figure 2.10, the olfactory bulb is located very close to all parts of the limbic system including the amygdala. That means that the aromatic molecules have a close connection to the emotional processing part of the limbic system and explains why the smell of hot chocolate makes you feel comforted and secure and may remind you of Grandma's kitchen in the winter. On a scientific level, mitral cells in the olfactory bulb, depicted in Figure 2.11, carry the output signals to the olfactory cortex in the brain, so that conscious perception of the aroma can take place.

Figure 2.12 indicates that axons of mitral cells in the olfactory bulb project into the primary olfactory cortex which connects to the limbic system, but some mitral cells connect directly to the amygdala (Kevetter and Winans 1981). Through its connections to the orbitofrontal cortex and thalamus, the amygdala plays a crucial role in ANS regulation and the stress response.

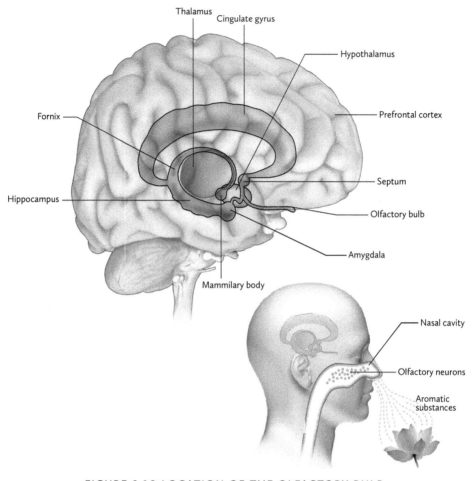

FIGURE 2.10 LOCATION OF THE OLFACTORY BULB.
Source: Baldwin A, 2020. Reiki in Clinical Practice: A Science-Based Guide. Handspring Publishing, Figure 5.2.

Sensory information from a calming aromatic oil, such as lavender, will dampen the response of the amygdala, impairing the "fight or flight" response, and enhancing the "rest and digest," or vagal response, reducing heart rate and increasing HRV. In fact, the degree of connectivity of the amygdala with the prefrontal cortex is directly related to HRV (Sakaki *et al.* 2016), which is the variation in time between heartbeats produced by changes in sympathetic and parasympathetic activities. A high HRV reflects a heart that is adaptable and responsive to second-by-second changes in the body's needs. If HRV, and its para-sympathetic component, root mean square of successive differences (RMSSD), both increase in response to inhaling lavender essential oil, this indicates that lavender aromatherapy is having a relaxing effect by activating the vagus nerve.

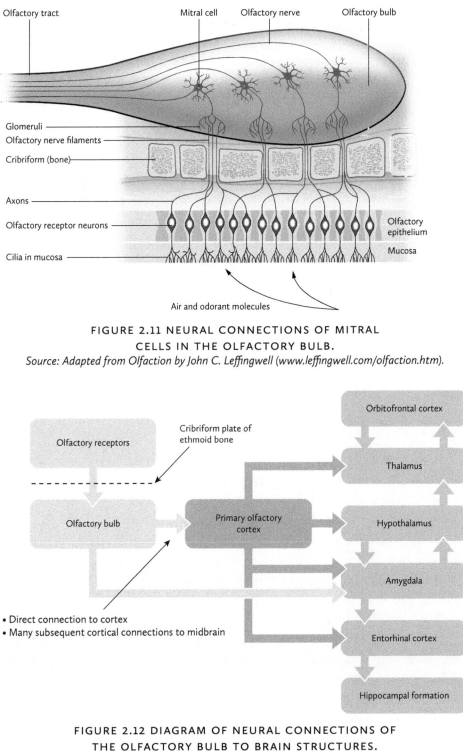

FIGURE 2.11 NEURAL CONNECTIONS OF MITRAL CELLS IN THE OLFACTORY BULB.
Source: Adapted from Olfaction by John C. Leffingwell (www.leffingwell.com/olfaction.htm).

FIGURE 2.12 DIAGRAM OF NEURAL CONNECTIONS OF THE OLFACTORY BULB TO BRAIN STRUCTURES.
Source: Used by permission of Jonathan Pillow. http://pillowlab.princeton. edu/teaching/sp2022/slides/Lec20_Olfaction_Chap14.pdf.

Evidence that aromatherapy increases vagal tone

Peer-reviewed scientific studies indicate that aromatherapy can produce a short-term relaxing effect on the ANS. A review of 16 randomized, controlled trials to test effects of aromatherapy on people with anxiety indicated a positive effect on their symptoms in most cases, especially on participants exhibiting higher levels of psychological distress (Lee *et al.* 2011). Although not a direct measure of vagal tone, a reduction in anxiety reflects a decrease in arousal away from the "fight or flight" response and towards the parasympathetic, or "rest and digest," response. The problem with these studies was that they relied on self-assessment of anxiety symptoms rather than on objective measures such as heart rate, blood pressure and HRV, and so were more subject to bias. For example, participants may react, either consciously or unconsciously, in a manner that they think the investigator wants, rather than responding naturally.

For relaxation, lavender is a popular choice of aromatic essential oil, and its medicinal properties have been noted in the British Pharmacopoeia for about 250 years. In a recent review of 21 controlled trials of lavender aromatherapy, the average stress score of the groups of people receiving lavender was significantly lower than that for the control groups (Ghavami *et al.* 2022). The authors concluded that "the use of lavender can be considered as a part of stress management programs, especially in student groups." However, once again the analysis relied on self-assessment of stress and anxiety symptoms rather than on objective measures.

Some published studies have used objective measures in assessing the relaxation effect of lavender aromatherapy in terms of its effects on vagal tone. For example, when lavender aromatherapy was given to 20 healthy volunteers, they experienced significant decreases in blood pressure, heart rate and skin temperature, which are all objective measures of a decrease in autonomic arousal (Sayorwan *et al.* 2012). In terms of their mood, those in the lavender oil group judged themselves to be more active, fresher and more relaxed than participants just inhaling base oil.

In another investigation, inhalation of lavender for 20 minutes twice a week for 12 weeks increased HRV and vagal tone compared to baseline values in 34 midlife women with insomnia compared to the control group of 33 women who only received health education concerning sleep hygiene (Chien *et al.* 2012). The women receiving aromatherapy also experienced a significant improvement in sleep quality after the intervention. This study directly shows that lavender aromatherapy works by stimulating the vagus nerve, because not only did HRV increase, but also the parasympathetic component of HRV, RMSSD, increased. It was hoped that the aromatherapy would have a long-term benefit, meaning that the vagal stimulation would persist between sessions, but the baseline values of HRV and RMSSD, measured four and 12 weeks after the start of aromatherapy, did not increase. Even so, the baseline very low frequency (VLF) contribution to HRV measured at four weeks was significantly higher than the initial baseline value in the experimental group. This is important because previous research has shown that sympathetic neural activity decreases the VLF band, and vagal activity increases the VLF band (Akselrod and Gorodon 1981).

Another review of 22 randomized, controlled studies to test the efficacy of lavender aromatherapy in relieving anxiety and its physiological manifestations showed that inhaling lavender oil reduced self-assessed anxiety as well as systolic blood pressure, heart rate and salivary cortisol (stress hormone) concentration (Kang *et al.* 2019). It was suggested that lavender aromatherapy be included in programs to manage anxiety in patients across diverse healthcare settings.

In summary, I think that there is already convincing evidence that lavender aromatherapy is effective in activating the vagus nerve to reduce stress and anxiety. Further research is needed to determine whether it can produce lasting effects.

CASE STUDY: Aromatherapy releases tension and anxiety
Norah Dykema, Energy Healer, Spiritual Teacher,
Practical Mystic (Norah@norahd.com)

My client arrived experiencing a high level of anxiety, describing it as a "ten" on a scale from one to ten, with one being the lowest level. She seemed scattered. She commented on the room, saying it was beautifully furnished and that she especially liked the plush, modern, turquoise-colored couch and the gold-colored chaise longue. I asked her to participate in an aromatherapy exercise to see if it would help her. She seated herself in a reclining position on the gold chaise longue and smelled "Stress Away" essential oil blend formulated by Young Living, out of the bottle. My client breathed it in deeply through her nose three times and immediately experienced a release of "an air bubble" (client's words) shooting out of her left shoulder and another out of her right foot. Her body language became more congruent with her feelings as she became more relaxed with me. She started talking about the reasons for her anxiety, and her eyes filled with tears as she spoke about why she had come for help. Her hands were coming up to shoulder level, palms upturned, indicating her frustration while describing her situations. Her voice would crack at times, and she was holding back from fully crying.

After a few minutes, she took three more deep sniffs from the bottle. She relaxed more and was able to feel her left ear opening up. A spot on the top of her head opened, and she felt more openings of flow in her shoulders and left side of her neck. After a few more minutes, she took three more sniffs. She began to feel "sleepy" (client's word) but noted this was because there was so much stress leaving her. I asked her to share where her level of stress and anxiety was at this point, which was at about 15 minutes in, and she noted it was down to a "four" and was starting to feel an effect hitting her heart area.

An opening had occurred that was moving some "stuck bad energy" (client's words) from her heart, and she was very surprised and decided to relax even more as she noticed this helped her "feel the path of aromatherapy working on her" (client's words). She began to feel a "widening" of energy open up in the left side of her neck, as if it were expanding. She felt "happier and hopeful" (client's words) as she had been struggling with some upsetting events. Her head was "clearing" and she said she was feeling "so much better" and her "mood" of anxiety had dropped to a "two." She noted that there were arteries and veins opening and that she could feel her energy was definitely being "moved in a healthy way" (client's words) for her.

My client was noticeably calm and happier after the aromatherapy. And she commented that she was "feeling hopeful." I felt she was a little giddy about having felt so much better. She was excited about our session. All of this took 24 minutes.

Stress Away Blend is a gentle fragrant blend that helps with normal, everyday stress, improves mental response, restores equilibrium, promotes relaxation, and lowers hypertension. Ingredients: copaiba, lime, cedarwood, vanilla, ocotea, and lavender.

To order Stress Away through Norah, please visit www.youngliving.com, use Referral ID 1253189. Stress Away comes in a 15 ml bottle or in a 10 ml roll-on bottle.

VAGAL STIMULATION WITH MASSAGE

As I described previously, the spinal accessory nerve is a motor nerve embedded in the sternocleidomastoid muscles on each side of the neck as well as the trapezius muscles on top of the shoulders. When moderate pressure is applied to the area between these muscles with twisting or stroking motions during massage (Figure 2.13), the spinal accessory nerve is activated.

The spinal accessory nerve is one part of the accessory nerve, which also has a cranial part. The spinal part of the accessory nerve connects to the spinal accessory nucleus and the cranial part to the vagus nerve (Bordoni *et al.* 2022) which joins up with the nucleus ambiguus. The anatomy of the two components of the accessory nerve and their connections to the spinal nucleus and nucleus ambiguus are shown in Figure 2.14.

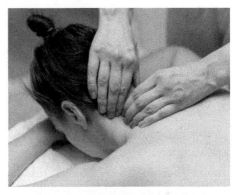

FIGURE 2.13 ACTIVATING THE SPINAL ACCESSORY NERVE WITH MASSAGE. *Source: Freepik.com.*

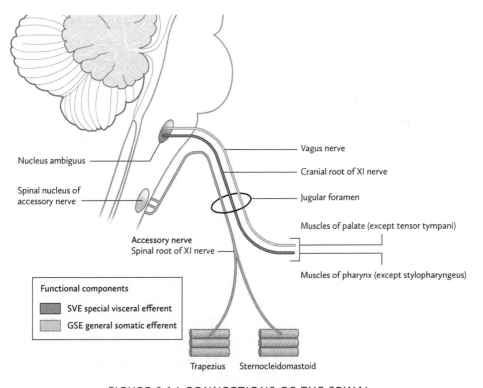

FIGURE 2.14 CONNECTIONS OF THE SPINAL ACCESSORY NERVE TO BRAIN STEM NUCLEI. *Source: Adapted from Anatomy Made Simple. Anatomy QA. Accessory Nerve.*

The anatomy of the spinal accessory nerve and its proximity to the vagus nerve raises the possibility that massage of the neck and shoulders not only activates the spinal accessory nerve but also influences the signaling of the nucleus ambiguus. If the nucleus ambiguus is stimulated, it provides parasympathetic output to the vagus nerve and coronary branch, increasing vagal tone to the heart, decreasing heart rate and shifting one away from "fight or flight" response and over to "rest and digest."

Evidence that massage of neck and shoulders increases vagal tone

The most convincing evidence that massage of the base of the head, neck and shoulders can increase vagal tone comes from a study in which 60 healthy women were randomly assigned to one of the following ten-minute procedures: (1) a vagus nerve targeted massage, (2) a soft shoulder massage, or (3) a resting control group (Meier *et al.* 2020). While the aim of the targeted massage was to maximally activate the vagus nerve by putting moderate pressure on the head/neck area, the soft massage was more of a "feel-good" massage, emphasizing the psychological and well-being components and lightly stimulating the back/shoulder area.

All three protocols did help participants relax as indicated by increases in their high frequency HRV which reflects parasympathetic stimulation, and decreases in their subjective stress levels. However, statistical analysis showed that both types of massage had significantly improved outcomes compared to the rest control group. These results indicate that although rest alone did increase vagal tone, massage was significantly more effective. The authors concluded that regular soft tissue massage of the shoulders improved vagal tone and so vagus nerve targeted massage may not be necessary. They recommended adding in a massage of the neck and shoulders once a week is a simple intervention to improve HRV, and thus vagal tone.

Another study that was performed on 30 young, healthy men and women who were randomly assigned to either a 20-minute massage or a rest period produced similar results (Delaney *et al.* 2002). In this case, the type of massage applied to the neck and trapezius muscle region was myofascial trigger point therapy which combines a variety of massage strokes with deeper more focused pressure at myofascial trigger points. Trigger points are small discrete hyperirritable areas within a taut band of muscular tissue or fascia.

Heart rate variability, blood pressure and self-assessment of emotional state and muscle tension were recorded before and after the intervention. Following the massage therapy, there were significant decreases in heart rate and blood pressure. Analysis of HRV revealed a significant increase in parasympathetic activity in terms of increases in high frequency HRV and RMSSD. Similar to the study with lavender aromatherapy (Akselrod and Gorodon 1981), HRV in the very low frequency (VLF) range was also increased, which is reflective of increased vagal tone. Additionally, both muscle tension and emotional state were significantly improved. There were no changes for the control group.

Massage of the neck and back for 25 minutes also improved vagal tone in 25 healthy children (Bayo-Tallon *et al.* 2019) as measured by increases in high frequency HRV and RMSSD. The RMSSD results persisted two weeks later. These improvements were not seen when the children were measured before and after a 25-minute rest-only period three months later. In a second group of children who received manual cranial therapy rather than massage, the benefits lasted for up to three weeks later.

In summary, I think that there is convincing evidence that massage of the neck and shoulder area is effective at stimulating the vagus nerve, resulting in a shift to a relaxed, parasympathetic state. Similar to aromatherapy, further research is needed to determine whether this type of massage can produce lasting effects on the ANS.

CASE STUDY: Multi-disciplinary medical massage

Gary Olsen, LMT, Mechanotherapist, Tucson Family
Wellness (gary@tucsonfamilywellness.com)

This is a review of vagus nerve treatment in a multi-disciplinary medical massage practice for a patient who had been in a car crash. We used massage, breathwork and The Work of Byron Katie.

A 35-year-old busy professional and mom came into my office. She had been referred for massage after a car crash she had been in a few months prior. She had been getting great care with chiropractic and physical therapy. She had come to a point where she was no longer progressing in her recovery as fast as she had been. I asked her how driving was for her these days after the crash. She had a big reaction, raising her hands and arms and saying in a much louder voice, "It is horrible! I have so much anxiety driving." She reported that whenever she drives now, while at most intersections, she is expecting to be hit by another car.

It was easy to see the hyper-alert panic reaction in her body as she talked about seeing cars that she thought would crash into her and her children.

She had a significant amount of tension in her jaw, neck, shoulders, chest and diaphragm. We did treatment with massage therapy, a breathwork practice (Tong Len) and questioning the thoughts identified (The Work of Byron Katie).

Massage therapy addressed areas of the body from her neck through her diaphragm and hip flexors. This helped her feel the tension and release into a deep relaxation state. We used trigger point massage, myofascial stretching and gentle Swedish massage. The massage helped her feel where her body was holding on in resistance. Gentle massage helped her release the resistance.

We did the Tong Len breathwork in the sessions as well. Tong Len is a Tibetan Buddhist meditation practice that is known as "giving and taking or sending and receiving." On the inhale, you take in the pain and suffering of yourself and others, and on the exhale, you give space, compassion and healing to yourself and others. This practice is great for gently moving directly through anxiety and all the body tension and pain reaction. This practice directly addresses resistance to anxiety in a very safe and gentle way. Because it gently moves through anxiety, the energetic charge is gone. She was empowered to do this on her own in a very quick way. Great opportunities to do this practice are just before and after driving.

The Work of Byron Katie helped her identify and question thoughts like "They are going to hit us." This work slows down that moment of seeing the car. It gave her the chance to see for real if it was true to her in that moment that "they are going to hit us." She got to experience how she reacts when believing this story. All the body tension and pain that we were working through came up when believing the thought. It was all connected and perfectly mirrored. Who was she without this thought? Without the story of "they are going to hit us," who was she?

Notice that with all these techniques we move gently and intentionally through pain, tension and anxiety. We acknowledge and experience the activation of stress on the vagus nerve and all its outcomes. We get to integrate the survival state and come to the clarity of being supported now. Coming to peace now is available. Will you receive it?

The patient reported great results from the first session. In her third session, she came in and stated she was complete with her recovery. She reported she was fully recovered, peaceful and grateful. Imagine how much money this saved the insurance company paying for all of her treatment.

REFERENCES

Akselrod S and Gorodon D, 1981. Power spectrum analysis of heart rate fluctuation: a quantitative probe of beat-to-beat cardiovascular control. *Science*. 213: 220–222.

Arai YC, Sakakima Y, Kawanishi J *et al.*, 2013. Auricular acupuncture at the "shenmen" and "point zero" points induced parasympathetic activation. *Evid Based Complement Alternat Med*. 2013: 945063. doi: 10.1155/2013/945063.

Baldry PE, 1993. *Acupuncture, Trigger Points and Musculoskeletal Pain*. Edinburgh: Churchill Livingstone.

Bayo-Tallon V, Esquirol-Caussa J, Pamias-Massana M *et al.*, 2019. Effects of manual cranial therapy on heart rate variability in children without associated disorders: translation to clinical practice. *Complementary Therapies in Clinical Practice*. 36: 125–141. doi: 10.1016/j.ctcp.2019.06.008.

Beukeboom CJ, Langeveld D and Tanja-Dijkstra K, 2012. Stress-reducing effects of real and artificial nature in a hospital waiting room. *J Altern Complement Med*. 18(4): 329–333. doi: 10.1089/acm.2011.0488.

Bivens RE, 2000. *Acupuncture, Expertise and Cross-Cultural Medicine*. Manchester: Palgrave.

Boehmer AA, Georgopoulos S, Nagel J *et al.*, 2020. Acupuncture at the auricular branch of the vagus nerve enhances heart rate variability in humans: an exploratory study. *Heart Rhythm O2*. 1(3): 215–221. doi: 10.1016/j.hroo.2020.06.001.

Bordoni B, Reed RR, Tadi P *et al.*, 2022. Neuroanatomy, Cranial Nerve 11 (Accessory). In: StatPearls [Internet]. Treasure Island (FL): StatPearls Publishing. www.ncbi.nlm.nih.gov/books/NBK507722.

Butt FM, Albusoda A, Farmer AD and Aziz Q, 2020. The anatomical basis for transcutaneous auricular vagus nerve stimulation. *J Anat*. 236: 588–611.

Cerrato PL, 1998. Aromatherapy: is it for real? *RN Journal of Nursing*. 61(6): 51–52.

Chien L-W, Cheng SL and Liu CF, 2012. The effect of aromatherapy on autonomic nervous system in midlife women with insomnia. *Evid Based Complementary Alternat Med*. 2012: 740813. doi: 10.1155/2012/740813.

Cui J, Wang S, Ren J, Zhang J and Jing J, 2017. Use of acupuncture in the USA: changes over a decade (2002–2012). *Acupunct Med*. 35(3): 200–207. doi: 10.1136/acupmed-2016-011106.

Delaney JPA, Leong KS, Watkins A and Brodie D, 2002. The short-term effects of myofascial trigger point massage therapy on cardiac autonomic tone in healthy subjects. *Journal of Advanced Nursing*. 37(4): 364–371.

Dimond EG, 1971. Acupuncture anesthesia. Western medicine and Chinese traditional medicine. *JAMA*. 218(10): 1558–1563.

Garcia-Diaz DE, Jimenez-Montufar LL, Guevara-Guzman R *et al.*, 1988. Olfactory and visceral projections to the nucleus of the solitary tract. *Physiology & Behavior*. 44(4–5): 619–624. doi: 10.1016/0031-9384(88)90327-7.

Ghavami T, Kazeminia M and Rajati F, 2022. The effect of lavender on stress in individuals: a systematic review and meta-analysis. *Complementary Therapies in Medicine*. 68: 102832. doi: 10.1016/j.ctim.2022.102832.

Hao JJ and Mittelman M, 2014. Acupuncture: past, present, and future. *Glob Adv Health Med*. 3(4): 6–8. doi: 10.7453/gahmj.2014.042.

Hornik J, 1984. Subjective vs. objective time measures: a note on the perception of time in consumer behaviour. *Journal of Consumer Research*. 11: 614–618.

International Federation of Aromatherapists, 2023. History of aromatherapy. Available from: https://ifaroma.org/en_GB/home/public_employers/explore_aromatherapy/essential-oils/history-aromatherapy.

Kang H-J, Nam ES, Lee Y and Kim M, 2019. How strong is the evidence for the anxiolytic efficacy of lavender? Systematic review and meta-analysis of randomized controlled trials. *Asian Nursing Research*. 13: 295–305.

Kaniusas E, Kampusch S, Tittgemeyer M *et al.*, 2019. Current directions in the auricular vagus nerve stimulation I – a physiological perspective. *Front Neurosci.* 13: 854. doi: 10.3389/fnins.2019.00854.

Karst M, Wintherhalter M, Munte S *et al.*, 2007. Auricular acupuncture for dental anxiety: a randomized controlled trial. *Anesth Analg.* 104: 295–300.

Kevetter GA and Winans SS, 1981. Connections of the corticomedial amygdala in the golden hamster. I. Efferents of the "vomeronasal amygdala." *J Comp Neurol.* 197(1): 81–98. doi: 10.1002/cne.901970107.

Kirchhof-Glazier D, n.d. Acupuncture: modern interest in an ancient technique. Huntingdon Health and Wellness Association. Available from: www.hhwa.org/complementary-modern-modalities/0u3zfyh63y8wgcyz1tzrb5xu8mqz46.

Lee YL, Wu Y, Tsang HWH *et al.*, 2011. A systematic review on the anxiolytic effects of aromatherapy in people with anxiety symptoms. *Journal of Alternative and Complementary Medicine.* 17(2): 101–108. www.liebertpub.com/doi/10.1089/acm.2009.0277.

Lehrner J, Marwinski G, Lehr S *et al.*, 2005. Ambient odors of orange and lavender reduce anxiety and improve mood in a dental office. *Physiology & Behavior.* 86(1–2): 92–95. doi: 10.1016/j.physbeh.2005.06.031.

Masaoka Y, Takayama M, Yajima H *et al.*, 2013. Analgesia is enhanced by providing information regarding good outcomes associated with an odor: placebo effects in aromatherapy? *Evidence Based Complementary and Alternative Medicine.* Volume 2013, Article ID 921802. doi: 10.1155/2013/921802.

Meier M, Unternaehrer E, Dimitroff SJ, *et al.*, 2020. Standardized massage interventions as protocols for the induction of psychophysiological relaxation in the laboratory: a block randomized, controlled trial. *Sci Rep.* 10(1):14774. doi: 10.1038/s41598-020-71173-w.

Miller DW, Roseen EJ, Stone JAM *et al.*, 2021. Incorporating acupuncture into American healthcare: initiating a discussion on implementation science, the status of the field, and stakeholder considerations. *Global Advances in Health and Medicine.* 10: 21649561211042574. doi: 10.1177/21649561211042574.

NICE, 2020. Chronic pain: assessment and management. Available from: www.nice.org.uk/guidance/ng193/documents/evidence-review-7.

NICE, 2021. Guideline [NG193]. Chronic pain (primary and secondary) in over 16s: assessment of all chronic pain and management of chronic primary pain. Available from: www.nice.org.uk/guidance/NG193.

NIH, 1997. Acupuncture. Consensus Statement. 15(5): 1-34.

Reston J, 1971. Now, about my operation in Peking. *The New York Times.* July 26, 1971; 1: 6.

Sakaki M, Yoo HJ, Nga L *et al.*, 2016. Heart rate variability is associated with amygdala functional connectivity with MPFC across younger and older adults. *Neuroimage.* 39: 44–52. doi: 10.1016/j.neuroimage.2016.05.076.

Sayorwan W, Siripornpanich V, Piriyapunyaporn T *et al.*, 2012. The effects of lavender oil inhalation on emotional states, autonomic nervous system, and brain electrical activity. *J Med Assoc Thai.* 95(4): 598–606.

Sok SR and Kim KB, 2005. Effects of auricular acupuncture on insomnia in Korean elderly. *Taehan Kanho Hakhoe Chi.* 35: 1014–1024.

Statista, 2022. Essential oils market worldwide: statistics & facts. Available from: www.statista.com/topics/5174/essential-oils/#dossierKeyfigures.

UK Health Centre, n.d. Acupuncture guide. Available from: www.healthcentre.org.uk/acupuncture.

Usichenko TI, Hua K, Cummings M *et al.*, 2022. Auricular stimulation for preoperative anxiety – a systematic review and meta-analysis of randomized controlled clinical trials. *Journal of Clinical Anesthesia.* 76: 110581. doi.org/10.1016/j.jclinane.2021.110581.

Wang SM, Peloquin C and Kain ZN, 2001. The use of auricular acupuncture to reduce preoperative anxiety. *Anesth Analg.* 93: 1178–1180.

White A and Ernst E, 2004. A brief history of acupuncture. *Rheumatology.* 43(5): 662–663. doi.org/10.1093/rheumatology/keg005.

CHAPTER 3

Laryngeal Branches

SINGING AND CHANTING

INTRODUCTION

To be able to speak, sing and chant, three systems need to work together: the laryngeal nerves, the laryngeal muscles and movement of the vocal folds as they respond to exhaled air. In this chapter, we will first describe the anatomy of these three systems in enough detail to explain how they function in unison to produce voice. Then we will clarify the mechanisms by which singing and chanting stimulate the vagus nerve, paying attention to the roles played by vibration of the vocal folds and to respiration. Finally, we will focus on how chanting affects the ANS, including the significance of the type of sound enunciated, the repetition frequency and the importance of people being together in a group. The principles will be illustrated by a case study of yogic chanting.

When you prepare to sing or chant, the brain sends a signal via the laryngeal branches of the vagus nerve to the muscles in the larynx, or voice box. As a result, these muscles open your voice box so that the vocal cords, or *folds* as they are more accurately called, are contacted by the air you are exhaling from your lungs through your larynx. The vocal folds vibrate, and vibration causes sound. The vibration of the vocal folds stimulates receptors in the laryngeal muscles which send signals back to the brain stem through sensory fibers in the laryngeal branches. Because the laryngeal branches connect to the vagus nerve, this nerve becomes stimulated. In this way, singing increases vagal tone, leading to a shift from the sympathetic "fight or flight" response to the parasympathetic "rest and digest" response. The pulmonary branches of the vagus nerve are also stimulated during singing or chanting because attention to the breath is a key component of these activities. So, the relaxation effect of singing and chanting happens in two separate ways, the long exhalation through the larynx and the vibration of the vocal folds.

People often sing when they are by themselves in the shower, and they find it pleasurable. Why does singing in the shower make one feel relaxed and even happy and confident? The feelings of happiness you experience as you sing in the shower may be related to the accompanying increase in the amplitude of your heart rate variability (HRV) and to the shift in its oscillatory frequency spectrum that signals an enhanced parasympathetic contribution from the vagus nerve (Bernardi *et al.* 2017).

As will be described later in this chapter, second-by-second changes in HRV are signalled from the heart to the brain's limbic system through the ANS. On receiving this information, the amygdala recognizes the emotional significance of the changes in HRV associated with singing in the shower. It has learned that a particular frequency oscillation pattern arising from a rhythmic shifting between sympathetic and parasympathetic stimulation reflects your own personal version of the "happy" state. Your heart is sending the amygdala this "happy" signal as you sing. The amygdala passes that information on to the prefrontal cortex or thinking part of the brain. In this way, you become consciously aware that singing in the shower makes you feel happy. A possible reason for the extra confidence you may feel as you sing in the shower is that your voice sounds so strong and hearty. Inside a shower, your voice bounces back and forth off the walls and other hard surfaces so you hear not only your voice as it is but also the echoes, or reverberation as the sound bounces off the walls.

ANATOMY OF LARYNGEAL NERVES AND MUSCLES

How do the laryngeal branches of the vagus complex operate the laryngeal muscles so that they open and close the vocal folds? First, we need to study the anatomy of the nerves. The left and right superior laryngeal nerves each split into the external laryngeal nerve and the internal laryngeal nerve (Figure 3.1). The *internal* branches are *sensory* and supply sensory fibers to the mucosa, or moist inner lining of the larynx, or voice box, above the vocal folds. The *external* laryngeal nerves are *motor* nerves and are the source of motor innervation to the cricothyroid muscle. This means that they send impulses from the nucleus ambiguus to the cricothyroid muscle of the larynx which tilts the thyroid forward to help tense the vocal folds.

The *inferior recurrent* laryngeal nerves pass along each side of the trachea, or windpipe, and innervate the larynx where the vocal folds are located. They are mixed nerves with both sensory and motor fibers. As can be seen in Figure 3.1, the left nerve loops under the aortic arch and then travels upward to the larynx. The right nerve (not shown) loops under the right subclavian artery before traveling upwards.

These nerves are called "recurrent" because they move in the opposite direction to the nerve they branch from – in this case, the vagus nerve. The sensory fibers transmit sensory information from the mucous membranes that lie beneath the lower surface of the vocal folds in the larynx to the nucleus solitarius located in the brain stem. The motor fibers send instructions from the nucleus ambiguus in the brain stem to the intrinsic muscles of the larynx that are responsible for opening, closing and changing the tension of your vocal folds. Without the inferior recurrent laryngeal nerves and the muscles that they serve, you would be unable to speak, let alone sing and chant.

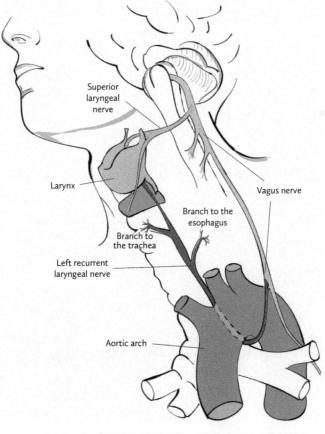

FIGURE 3.1 ANATOMY OF THE LARYNGEAL NERVES.
Source: Wikimedia Commons, CC BY-SA 3.0.

The posterior cricoarytenoid muscles, despite their unwieldy name, are very important because they are the only muscles that open the vocal folds (Branca-tisano *et al.* 1984). When these muscles contract in response to signals from the inferior recurrent laryngeal nerves, this causes the arytenoid cartilages to rotate and open the glottis. The glottis is a slit-like opening on the floor of the pharynx, which controls airflow in and out of the respiratory passages and opens directly into larynx (or voice box) where the vocal folds are located. When the glottis opens, this separates the vocal folds and helps the other intrinsic muscles to lengthen the vocal folds, allowing the passage of air during inhalation and exhalation. The vocal folds vibrate, and sound is produced. For this reason, the posterior cricoarytenoid muscle is the most important muscle in the larynx for respiration and speech.

THE VOICE MECHANISM: VOCAL FOLDS

Before we explore the voice mechanism, it is important to note that the most important function of your larynx is to protect your lungs from accidental influx of food and water. The larynx is positioned just above the airway to the lungs, and the vocal folds form a valve that closes tightly to protect this airway, also known as the windpipe, or trachea. When you swallow, the vocal folds come together so that the glottis closes tightly, preventing saliva and food from passing into the trachea instead of entering the esophagus, or gullet. Figure 3.2 shows how these structures are arranged.

The larynx has three main parts:

- supraglottis, the area above the vocal folds
- glottis, the middle area where the vocal folds are located
- subglottis, the area below the vocal folds that connects to the windpipe (trachea).

Voice is produced by the internal muscles of the larynx and the laryngeal nerves working together to open and close the vocal folds as each exhaled breath passes through the larynx or voice box. Lateral cricoarytenoid, thyroarytenoid, inter-arytenoid and cricothyroid muscles all act together to open the vocal folds, and the posterior cricoarytenoid muscle closes them. All these muscles are paired and are symmetrically arranged on the left and right sides of the larynx. All the internal muscles of the larynx receive their nerve supply from the recurrent laryngeal nerve except the cricothyroid, which is innervated by the external branch of the superior laryngeal nerve. Figure 3.3 shows the arrangement of some of these muscles as viewed from above the larynx.

The thyroarytenoid muscles are the muscles that form the vocal folds themselves (V-shape in Figure 3.3). They shorten the vocal folds by pulling the back end of the vocal folds (arytenoid end) toward the front end (thyroid end) as shown by the arrows. This causes them to vibrate more slowly because they are looser, thus lowering pitch. The thyroarytenoid muscles are also able to strengthen closure of the glottis. They help bring the vocal folds together and keep them together to resist the exhalation of air from the lungs. The other intrinsic muscles also work together to change the position, tension and pressure of the vocal folds. Figure 3.4 depicts the view from above the vocal folds, showing how they open and close.

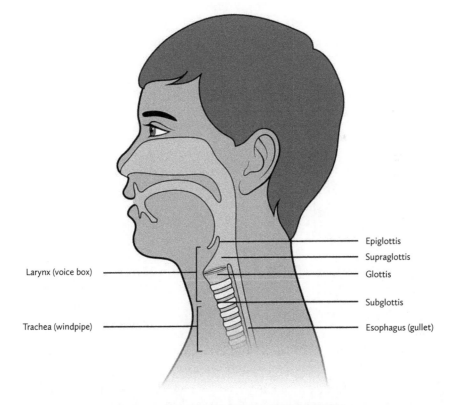

FIGURE 3.2 POSITION OF THE LARYNX.
Source: This image was produced by Macmillan Cancer Support and is reused with their permission.

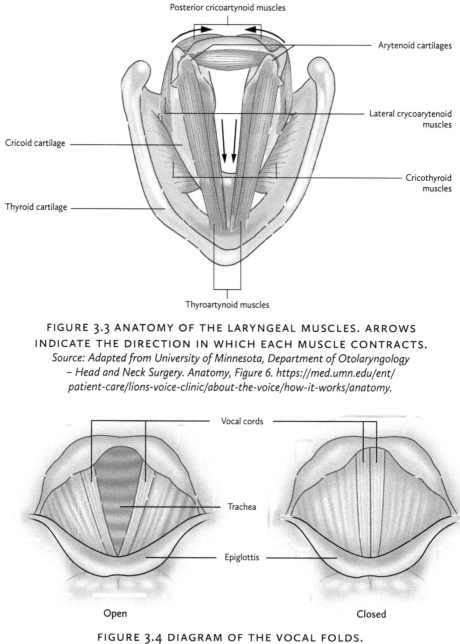

FIGURE 3.3 ANATOMY OF THE LARYNGEAL MUSCLES. ARROWS INDICATE THE DIRECTION IN WHICH EACH MUSCLE CONTRACTS.
Source: Adapted from University of Minnesota, Department of Otolaryngology – Head and Neck Surgery. Anatomy, Figure 6. https://med.umn.edu/ent/ patient-care/lions-voice-clinic/about-the-voice/how-it-works/anatomy.

FIGURE 3.4 DIAGRAM OF THE VOCAL FOLDS.
Source: Used by permission of Dysphonia International. https:// dysphonia.org/your-journey/how-voice-works/vocal-cords.

When we say that the vocal folds "vibrate," they do not actually vibrate like a string. Instead, small pulses of air from the lungs and diaphragm pass through the vocal folds, creating pressure changes within the vocal tract and producing sound. During the closed phase, the air pressure builds up below the vocal folds. When the glottis opens, the air rushes through the vocal folds, which begins the sound wave. The folds separate in a wave-like fashion, starting from the bottom and moving towards the top. The faster the vocal folds vibrate, the higher the pitch. Extremely slow vocal fold vibration is about 60 vibrations per second (Hz) and produces a low pitch. Extremely fast vocal fold vibration approaches 2000 Hz and produces a very high pitch. Only children and the highest sopranos can reach those extremely high pitches. In general, men's vocal folds vibrate at 85–155 Hz during normal speech, whereas the range for women is 165–255 Hz (Baken 2000).

HOW DO SINGING AND CHANTING STIMULATE THE VAGUS NERVE?

Movement of the vocal folds

As we learned in Chapter 2, auricular acupuncture causes sensory stimulation of nerves in the skin of the ear. Likewise, singing and chanting cause sensory changes in the larynx. For example, the uneven airflow passing through the glottis as you sing causes the intrinsic laryngeal muscles to stretch and relax, which stimulates stretch receptors in those muscles. The stretch receptor response is relayed through sensory nerve fibers of the internal laryngeal and inferior recurrent laryngeal nerve branches to the main vagus branch and then to the nucleus solitarius in the brain stem (see Figures 3.1 and 3.5). The nucleus solitarius then communicates to the nucleus ambiguus, and instructions are sent through the motor nerve fibers of the vagus nerve which connects to the external laryngeal and inferior recurrent laryngeal nerves. These instructions enable muscular adjustments so that the vocal folds keep at the intended length and tension to maintain a steady vocal pitch. As can be seen in Figure 3.5, if the vagal motor fibers are activated in this way, the stimulation will pass into the cardiac plexus through the coronary branches leading to the sinoatrial node of the heart. The vagal input results in reduced heart rate and increased HRV – in other words, relaxation. The mind-body is shifted to the parasympathetic, "rest and digest" state.

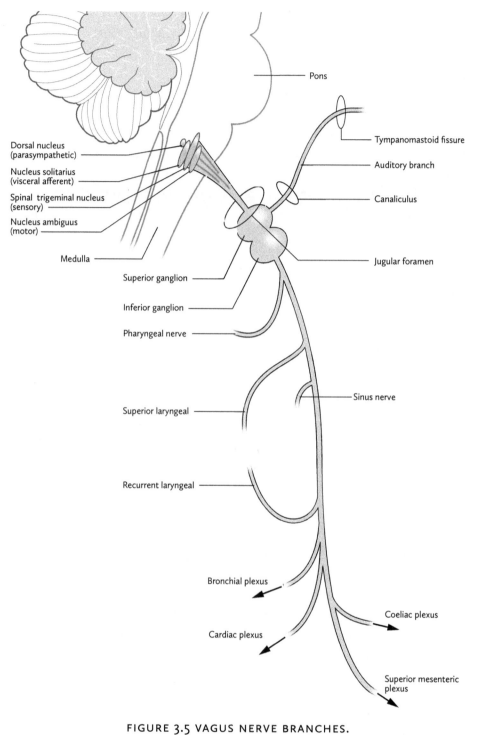

FIGURE 3.5 VAGUS NERVE BRANCHES.
*Source: Adapted from Anatomy and Physiology MCQs. http://cambridgequestions.
co.uk/displayquestion.aspx?id=535. © anatomymcqs.com.*

So, stimulation of the laryngeal nerve branches during singing and chanting leads to activation of the vagus nerve because the cranial nerves and vagal branches are all part of the same network, the ventral vagal system. One potential disadvantage of having a common neural network is noted as follows in a publication by Karemaker (2022):

> However, the problem in application of whole vagus nerve stimulation is the lack of specificity: there is no way to titrate the stimulation to an observable effect variable. All nerves in the bundle, incoming and outgoing, can be "hit," leading to side-effects which limit the intended application.

Gareth Ackland of University College London compares vagus stimulation to flipping on a light switch in one room of a house and discovering that this endows other rooms in the house with magical powers. "I'm not sure which room it's going to happen in, I'm not sure for how long and I'm not sure if, after a while, it's going to work or not," he says (Schwartz 2015). For this reason, it is important not only to think about the expected, desired effect of a certain vagal stimulation therapy, but also to consider what other extraneous reactions might be triggered and whether they will benefit the recipient. In the case of singing and chanting, two physiological processes are activated that both enhance vagal stimulation, which is what we want, so there is no need to worry. One is the movement of the vocal folds as described previously, and the other is the exhalation during respiration. Now we will consider the effect of those long exhales on the autonomic state while chanting "Om."

The long exhale

Use of the voice is built upon a foundation of respiration. Your breath is the power source for speaking, singing and chanting. The vagus nerve is also influenced by voluntary and involuntary cycles of respiration. When you inhale, the vagal activity is reduced and so your heart beats faster, but as you exhale, the vagus nerve is more fully engaged and your heart beats more slowly. The physiological mechanisms behind this response are quite complicated and will be explained more fully in Chapters 4 and 5.

If you breathe at five or six breaths per minute, which is about five seconds in and five seconds out, this differential effect on the vagus nerve is maximized. The average respiration rate for most people when they are at rest is between 12 and 15 breaths per minute. This means that you need to breathe slower than normal to fully engage the increased vagal activity and subsequent decreased heart rate associated with the exhale. It is very easy to test this for yourself. Just place the tips of the index and middle fingers of one hand on your other wrist under the thumb. You should be able to feel your pulse. Now breathe deeply and slowly and keep your attention on your pulse rate. You will find that as you inhale, your pulse is faster and more noticeable, and as you exhale, your pulse is slower and fainter. This coupling of heart rate to respiration is called respiratory sinus arrhythmia (RSA). Your heart rate varies exactly in phase with your breathing. The two systems are synchronized. This state is also known as "coherence."

The pattern of HRV associated with coherence is shown in Figure 3.6 (lower panel). The rhythmic change in heart rate is immediately apparent. If respiration rate is monitored simultaneously with HRV, the rise and fall in lung volume with each breath mirrors the rise and fall in heart rate in the coherent state. This phenomenon is illustrated in Chapter 4. The HRV pattern at a given moment is sent directly from the heart to the brain stem through the ANS and then to the limbic system and prefrontal cortex. If the HRV pattern is coherent you experience a soothing effect. On the other hand, the far less organized, incoherent HRV signal (Figure 3.6, upper panel), has the opposite result and can even impair brain function in several ways. Further details of the heart-brain link and how HRV can influence emotional regulation and cognitive abilities will be described in Chapter 4.

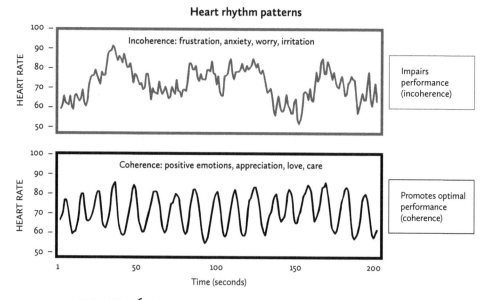

FIGURE 3.6 COHERENCE AND HEART RATE VARIABILITY.
Source: © 2013 HeartMath Institute. www.heartmath.org.

To shift the ANS balance even more to the parasympathetic side, you can exhale for a longer period compared to the inhale. For example, Dr Andrew Weil recommends the 4-7-8 breath for relaxation, in which you inhale for four seconds, hold your breath for seven seconds and exhale for eight seconds (www.drweil.com/health-wellness/body-mind-spirit/stress-anxiety/breathing-three-exercises). However, this type of breathing does not maximize HRV and RSA and it does not synchronize the inward and outward breaths with HRV. You will probably feel more relaxed compared to your normal breathing state, but you will not experience the other physiological and psychological benefits of coherence. For example, when respiration and HRV are synchronized (high RSA), there is evidence that the work done by the heart is minimized while maintaining healthy levels of blood gases (Ben-Tal *et al.* 2012). In addition, increased HRV, within the normal range, reflects a greater ability of the body to dynamically adjust to changing internal and external environments by allowing a healthy interaction between the sympathetic and parasympathetic branches of the ANS (Thayer *et al.* 2010).

Singing and especially chanting involve repetitive long exhales that cause vibration of the vocal folds. Do singing and chanting produce a coupling of respiration and heart rate and an increase in HRV? Studies show that for singing, the answer depends on the nature of the music – in other words, the tempo and phrases. A phrase is a single unit of music that makes complete musical sense when heard on its own, such as singing "Happy birthday to you" without singing the whole song. Vickhoff *et al.* (2013) showed that the effects of singing on HRV depend on the specific form of singing, with a mantra sung at a rhythm of six breaths/minute (0.1 Hz) yielding the maximum increase in HRV and RSA.

Interestingly another study showed that when priests recited the rosary and monks chanted mantras, their respiration rates fell naturally to five breaths per minute (0.1 Hz) (Bernardi *et al.* 2001). Olsson *et al.* (2013) demonstrated that group singing of slow songs resulted in slower heart rate and greater HRV compared to faster songs. Chanting appears to be even more effective at activating the vagus nerve than singing and will be discussed more fully in the next section.

WHY IS CHANTING ESPECIALLY EFFECTIVE FOR RELAXATION?

The sound of Om

The word "Om" is often chanted at the beginning of yoga classes. According to audio producer and yoga teacher Ainhoa Acosta, "Om" is a sacred Sanskrit word that means "All." It is not associated with any specific religion, but Hindu tradition believes it to be the cosmic sound that initiated the start of the universe. Although it appears to consist of one syllable, it forms three sounds because it is pronounced "a-u-m," reflecting the continuity of the past, present and future, or birth, life and death.

Ainhoa Acosta (2020) describes the physical sensations that are elicited by chanting "Om":

> At a physical level, the Aum syllable addresses the whole of the human sound instrument: we open the mouth ("a"), move the lips closer to each other ("u") and then close the mouth ("m"). This activates the larynx fully. "A" resonates in the stomach and chest, "u" in the throat and chest and "m" in the nasal cavity, skull, and brain. By chanting Aum we move the energy from the abdomen up to the brain. Those of us who chant Aum daily before our practice, feel how it helps us to calm our mind and clear our thoughts.

It has been suggested that chanting "Om" produces a vibratory sensation in the ears that spreads through the auricular branches of the vagus nerve, stimulating the vagal complex (Gangadhar *et al.* 2011). In this way, chanting takes advantage of three routes to vagal stimulation: the laryngeal nerves, the auricular nerves and through RSA.

Shirley Telles, a neurophysiologist and Director of Patanjali Research Foundation in Haridwar, India, helped conduct a study to determine whether there was anything specific about chanting the sound "Om," rather than some other word, that would shed light on the mind-body benefits. The researchers measured autonomic changes in participants who mentally repeated two syllables, one which was meaningful (Om) and the other, neutral (Telles *et al.* 1998). The results showed that participants experienced a decrease in heart rate and respiration rate when chanting both types of sounds compared to non-targeted thinking, indicating a relaxation response. However, only when chanting "Om" did they show an increase in skin conductance, which is associated with sweating and increased mental arousal. The authors speculated that the skin conductance reaction was caused by an increase in the attentional arousal of the participants because when reciting "Om," they perceived it as something significant compared to the neutral sound.

The concept associated with "Om" is the entirety of the universe. Subjects with longer meditation experience did not show this change, possibly because they had become used to the sound and it no longer engaged their attention in the same way. Instead, experienced meditators demonstrated an improved ability to receive and respond to information coming in through the senses. So, with long-term practice, chanting "Om" may do more than just help you relax by activating the vagus nerve; more subtle cognitive changes may also occur. With practice, the relaxation effect also improves. Inbaraj *et al.* (2022) showed that although naïve meditators showed a significant increase in the parasympathetic component of HRV after chanting "Om" for five minutes, experienced meditators came in with an already heightened vagal activity, which was further amplified after a five-minute chant. The magnitude of the increase in vagal activity after chanting was positively correlated with the number of years' experience in yoga.

How fast should you chant?

Surprisingly, there is very little information in the literature about the optimal speed with which one should chant "Om," or how long to take in enunciating each "Om." Some useful guidelines are provided by Mrs. Poornima Mandlik (Rishi Dharmasheela) from Yoga Vidya Gurukul. Yoga Vidya Gurukul has been recognized by AYUSH (Yoga and Ayurveda) ministry, Government of India, as the Leading Yoga Institution in India. Her instructions are shown in Boxes 3.1 and 3.2.

BOX 3.1 HOW TO CHANT OMKAR

AUM can be chanted slowly or quickly. Each method is as good as the other and you must experiment yourself to find out your own preference. If chanted quickly, then it is a powerful method to synchronize it with the heartbeat. In this manner you feel AUM resonating throughout the whole body in tune with the natural heart rate.

If AUM is chanted slowly, it can be made to last many seconds, depending on the capacity of the individual. There should be definite pronunciation of each of the syllables, "A," "U" and "M," with a gradual transition of one to another. "A" is pronounced as "a" in "palm," "U" is pronounced as "ooo," and "M" is pronounced as a humming sound by closing the lips "mmmmmmm." The sound of "A" should start at the navel, "U" from the chest and "M" from brain (head). The sound should be generated from the navel and taken up very slowly to the top of the head with the closing sound of "M." "A" is pronounced by opening the mouth slightly, without touching the tongue to the palates of the mouth, "U" is pronounced by opening the mouth in a beak shape, like whistling, the tongue touching the back of the lower teeth slightly, "M" is pronounced by closing the mouth and simply producing the humming sound (mmmmmmmm). All the three sounds should be continuous and in rhythm, like the water pouring continuously. Just like the ringing of a bell the sound and vibrations are heard for a long time, called "ninaad." In the same way AUM should be chanted, with the "M" sound leaving its vibration.

Source: Mrs Poornima Mandlik. www.yogapoint.com/mainstory/TopstoryContents/Om_Aum_mantra.htm.

BOX 3.2 PREPARATION FOR CHANTING OMKAR
Practice of Omkar chanting for 5 minutes

Please sit in a relaxed position, keep your spine erect and gently close your eyes.

Try to relax your whole body, relax your left hand from fingers to shoulder, relax your right hand from finger to shoulder.

Relax left foot from toes to waist; relax right foot from toes to waist.

Now concentrate on the front side of your body, abdomen, chest.

Concentrate on the back side of your body, neck muscles, spine, shoulders, upper back, lower back.

Now try to relax your face, chin, left cheek, right cheek, left eye, eye lid, eyeball, eyebrow, right eye, eye lid, eyeball, eyebrow, forehead, top of the head, back side of the head.

After relaxing the whole body, concentrate on your natural breathing for some time.

Start practicing deep breathing very slowly.

Inhale and exhale slowly and deeply...relax whole body again and again.

Try to increase the amount of oxygen with deep breathing, deep inhalation, deep exhalation.

After a few deep breaths concentrate on normal breathing.

Chant Aum (AUMMMMMM) for 5 minutes and finish with shanti path.

Om shanti shanti shanti.

*Source: Mrs Poornima Mandlik. www.yogapoint.com/
mainstory/TopstoryContents/Om_Aum_mantra.htm.*

Note the emphasis that Mrs. Poornima Mandlik places on deep, slow breathing when chanting "Om," indicating the importance of being in the coherent state. For that reason, I would recommend chanting at six cycles per minute for each "Om"; five seconds to breathe in and five seconds to chant "Om." That way, not only will you ensure a rhythmic, dependable activation of the vagus nerve with each breath, but you will maximize the resulting physiological and psychological benefits of being in the coherent ANS state.

Alone or together?

Singing and chanting by yourself is healthy for mind and body. You do not have to be in a group to reap the benefits. Your vocal folds vibrate and your breath flows as you sing and chant whether you are alone in the shower or on stage in a group at the Royal Albert Hall, but recent research suggests that singing in a group may add some more benefits compared to being solo.

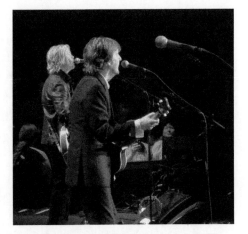

FIGURE 3.7 SINGING IN A ROCK GROUP AT THE ROYAL ALBERT HALL.

Good and Russo (2021) studied a group of eight healthy older adults from a community choir as they sang alone and together. The researchers deliberately chose to investigate singers who were in a low-stress, supportive environment. This is important in the context of providing a neutral baseline for determining whether singing is effective for increasing relaxation and improving mind-body health. Here we are not talking about reaching the perfect pitch in a professional performance, where the singing itself may act as a stressor, but singing and chanting for enjoyment.

The investigators chose older adults to participate in this study because older people may experience many challenges to their social and psychological well-being such as social isolation, loneliness and stress related to aging, and social activities like singing in a choir might help them with these issues. The question posed by the study was: "Does singing as a group reduce stress and improve mental health more than singing alone?" Participants completed a mood questionnaire and provided saliva samples for analysis of the stress hormone cortisol, and another hormone/neurotransmitter, oxytocin, before and after singing alone or together for 45-minute sessions.

Oxytocin is commonly known as the "bonding hormone" because it seems to help reinforce early attachment between mothers and their infants and bonding between romantic partners (Crockford *et al.* 2014). The two main physical functions of oxytocin are to stimulate uterine contractions in labor and childbirth and to stimulate contractions of breast tissue to aid in lactation after childbirth. In the last decade or so, oxytocin has attracted substantial research interest for its role in behavior and cognition, and that is probably why it was selected as an outcome parameter in this study. However, searching through the scientific literature reveals that the evidence for these effects has been mixed.

The results showed that both group and individual singing reduced salivary concentrations of the stress hormone, cortisol. A previous study demonstrated that when a group of professional singers sang in a low-stress environment, their salivary cortisol concentrations also decreased (Fancourt *et al.* 2015). Interestingly, when the same people sang during a live concert, their cortisol concentrations significantly increased. So, it is very important to consider the type of environment in which you sing or chant if you are doing so primarily to benefit your health and well-being, whether alone or in a group.

What about oxytocin? In contrast to the results with cortisol, only group singing significantly elevated oxytocin and mood scores. The more that oxytocin increased, the greater was the improvement in mood (the results are shown in Figure 3.8). Although individual singing can regulate stress, elevations in mood and oxytocin appear to be driven by social factors. Another investigation highlights the importance of how you are regarded within the group (de Dreu *et al.*

2011). The authors reported that oxytocin's social bonding effects are targeted at whomever a person perceives as part of their in-group.

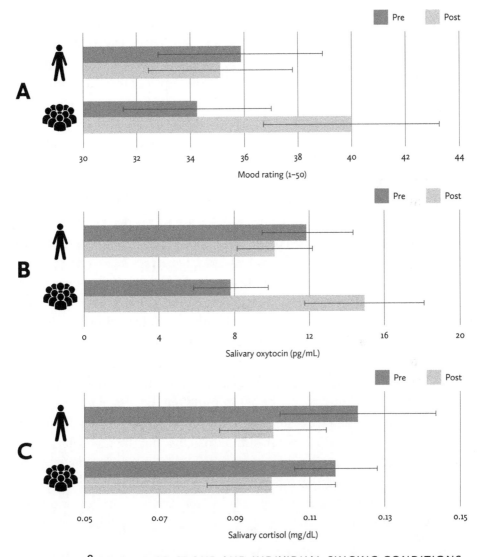

FIGURE 3.8 EFFECTS OF GROUP AND INDIVIDUAL SINGING CONDITIONS
ON THREE DIFFERENT OUTCOME VARIABLES: (A) MOOD IMPROVEMENTS,
(B) OXYTOCIN INCREASES AND (C) CORTISOL DECREASES.
Error bars represent one standard error.
Source: Arla Good and Frank A Russo, Psychology of Music. 50(4): 1340–1347, figure 1, copyright © 2022. Reprinted by Permission of SAGE Publications.

There is scientific evidence that singing or chanting in a group may produce physiological synchrony between participants based on HRV. If most of the participants are in the HRV coherent state in which respiration and heart rate are synchronized at a frequency close to six cycles per minute (0.1 Hz), the personal synchrony may extend to the whole group. Vickhoff et al. (2013) showed that when five singers sang regular song structures, or mantras, in unison, their heart rates increased and decreased simultaneously. This was also seen to some degree with humming during which participants breathed more slowly and deeply than usual. Baseline recordings show low depth of breathing, low HRV and no noticeable synchrony between participants. Singing a hymn produced complex results from which it was not possible to detect any obvious synchrony.

Similar results were found when non-expert singers sang in pairs (Ruiz-Blais et al. 2020). In this study, the authors were able to analytically separate out the RSA, or breathing component of the HRV coupling between pairs, and found that some coupling still remained when participants sang long notes. This suggested that some other mechanism, apart from RSA, was also involved in the coupling process, such as synchronization of vocal muscular action or perception of voice. Since the vagus nerve links the vocal folds, facial expressions and heart rate, it may be possible that the voice affects HRV through the ANS. One of the possible implications of HRV synchrony or entrainment between people is a potential role in bonding, by simultaneously affecting the psycho-physiological state of group members, but this needs to be supported by research.

In summary, singing and chanting are both very powerful methods for stimulating the vagus nerve as long as the focus is on vocalizing long notes, preferably with a rhythm of around six cycles per minute (0.1 Hz). The combination of movement of the vocal waves, vibration of the sound in the ears and slow rhythmic breathing makes a triple contribution to activating the vagus nerve. The effectiveness of these mechanisms is supported by rigorous scientific research. Singing or chanting in a group provides added benefits that are largely driven by social factors, as long as the environment is stress-free and the goal is to relax and enjoy the process.

CASE STUDY: The medicine of breath and chant

Tejpal Kaur, MA, MBA, Life Coach, Brennan Energy
Healer, Kundalini Yoga Teacher, Author,
Tejpal-Inspires (tejpal@tejpal-inspires.com)

As a Kundalini yoga teacher, I am part of tradition that offers many breath patterns and many chants. Both breath and chant train the mind to be more relaxed and more flexible. An untrained mind can be agitated, fixed on its position, and often looks for trouble.

Breath

Breath is one of the fastest ways to create a shift in a person's life. Breath, thought patterns and emotions are interrelated. When our breath changes, our emotions and thought patterns will automatically shift. If you are afraid, your breath will constrict; if you are angry, your breath will tighten; if you are grateful, your breath will be relaxed and so on. To understand the interdependence between breath, thought patterns and emotions, do the following breath exercise: inhale, exhale, hold the breath out and try to be worried or anxious. Most likely you will not be able to experience these emotions.

Many students who practice a three-minute breath practice will experience it as calming, clearing, grounding, or centering. The simple action of paying attention to the breath helps the mind to slow down, become quieter and more pliable. In the Kundalini yoga tradition, there is a breath for everything: strengthening your nervous system, balancing the right and left brain, clearing your energy field, healing your physical body, developing your intuition, clearing emotions from the past, and the list goes on. Most breath patterns are combined with a mantra (a word or phrase repeated in silence) and a mudra (a particular hand position) to enhance the healing potency of the breath.

Chant

In the yogic tradition, the universe or multiverse is built on sounds. The chant Om (pronounced A, U, M, silence) is an ongoing vibration in the universe; without this vibration, the universe would not exist. Everything is a vibration: our thoughts, our emotions, our physical organs, the clouds, the plants, etc.

Like breath work, chanting is also potent medicine for the mind, body and spirit. The art of chanting itself focuses on the exhale; you will not chant on the inhale. In some yogic traditions, the roof of the mouth is described to have 84 points of energy. When these points are stimulated with the tongue, the glandular system gets activated and chemical changes happen in the brain.

Chanting exists in many spiritual traditions. In fact, every culture carries unique sounds and chants to harmonize, unify the group and transcend individual needs – whether it is for spiritual purpose or war.

Chanting is always welcomed in a Kundalini yoga class. Whether students are struggling with stressful situations, challenging emotions or are simply tired, they can truly enjoy chanting. This does not depend on any musical or vocal abilities. Students feel transported to another field of reality; the music becomes a vibration in their body and mind. Every chant has a unique tempo: the melody, the mantra and the rhythm of the chant gives an opportunity for our whole system to become synchronized. Many people have shared that they feel the chant is chanting itself; they become one with everything without losing their sense of self. The mind then becomes spacious. Often, they will keep hearing the mantra throughout the day.

Chanting gives us an internal massage. Our mind becomes sensitive instead of objective; it does not operate in duality anymore. The mind, instead of contracting and objectifying, relaxes and expands our viewpoint and our experience. New pathways of communication and exchange of information are activated within us; we can now feel and see with our whole body. Our sensory system changes, and we now have a physical experience of the infinite in our finite bodies.

Some yogis have chosen to have a chant all night long in low volume to keep carrying them through the dream state; some choose to have chants ongoing in their house even when they leave their home to create a certain frequency of energy. Like breath patterns, there is a mantra and a chant for everything. Both breath and chant are powerful practices for experiencing grounding, inner stability, spaciousness and peace. A breath practice starts at the cellular level and then affects the mind; a chant simultaneously impacts the mind and the physical body.

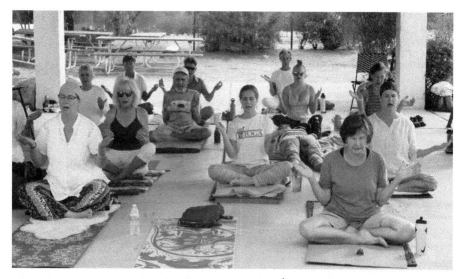

FIGURE 3.9 STUDENTS CHANTING IN TEJPAL'S KUNDALINI YOGA CLASS.

REFERENCES

Acosta A, 2020. The science and philosophy of om-aum. Available from: https://iyengaryogalon-don.co.uk/the-science-and-philosophy-of-om-aum.

Baken RJ, 2000. *Clinical Measurement of Speech and Voice*. 2nd edition. London: Taylor and Francis.

Ben-Tal A, Shamailov SS and Paton JF, 2012. Evaluating the physiological significance of respiratory sinus arrhythmia: looking beyond ventilation-perfusion efficiency. *J Physiol*. 590(8): 1989–2008. doi: 10.1113/jphysiol.2011.222422.

Bernardi L, Sleight P, Bandinelli G and Cencetti S, 2001. Effect of rosary prayer and yoga mantras on autonomic cardiovascular rhythms: comparative study. *BMJ*. 323(7327): 1446–1449.

Bernardi NF, Snow S, Peretz I *et al.*, 2017. Cardiorespiratory optimization during improvised singing and toning. *Sci Rep*. 7: 8113. doi: 10.1038/s41598-017-07171-2.

Brancatisano TP, Dodd DS and Engel LA, 1984. Respiratory activity of posterior cricoarytenoid muscle and vocal cords in humans. *Journal of Applied Physiology*. 57(4): 1143–1149. doi: 10.1152/jappl.1984.57.4.1143.

Crockford C, Deschner T, Ziegler TE and Wittig RM, 2014. Endogenous peripheral oxytocin measures can give insight into the dynamics of social relationships: a review. *Frontiers in Behavioral Neuroscience*. 8: 68. doi: 10.3389/fnbeh.2014.00068.

De Dreu CKW, Greer LL, Van Kleef GA and Handgraaf MJJ, 2011. Oxytocin promotes human ethrocentrism. Proceedings of the National Academy of Sciences. 108(4): 1262–1266. doi: 10.1073/pnas.1015316108.

Fancourt D, Aufegger L and Willliamon A, 2015. Low-stress and high-stress singing have contrasting effects on glucocorticoid response. *Frontiers of Psychology*. 6: 2015. doi: 10.3389/fpsyg.2015.01242.

Gangadhar B, Kalyani B, Venkatasubramanian G *et al.*, 2011. Neurohemodynamic correlates of "OM" chanting: a pilot functional magnetic resonance imaging study. *Int J Yoga*. 4: 3.

Good A and Russo FA, 2021. Changes in mood, oxytocin, and cortisol following group and individual singing: a pilot study. *Psychology of Music*. 50(4): 1340–1347. doi: 10.1177/03057356211042668.

Inbaraj G, Rao MR, Ram A *et al.*, 2022. Immediate effects of OM chanting on heart rate variability measures compared between experienced and inexperienced yoga practitioners. *Int J Yoga*. 15: 52–58.

Karemaker JM, 2022. The multibranched nerve: vagal function beyond heart rate variability. *Biological Psychology*. 172: 108378. doi: 10.1016/j.biopsycho.2022.108378.

Olsson E, Von Schéele B and Theorell T, 2013. Heart rate variability during choral singing. *Music and Medicine*. 5(1): 52–59.

Ruiz-Blais S, Orini M and Chew E, 2020. Heart rate variability synchronizes when non-experts vocalize together. *Frontiers in Physiology*. 11: 2020. doi: 10.3389/fphys.2020.00762.

Schwartz S, 2015. Viva vagus: wandering nerve could lead to range of therapies. ScienceNews. Available from: www.sciencenews.org/article/viva-vagus-wandering-nerve-could-lead-range-therapies.

Telles S, Nagarathna R and Nagendra HR, 1998. Autonomic changes while mentally repeating two syllables: one meaningful and the other neutral. *Indian J Physiol Pharmacol*. 42(1): 57–63.

Thayer JF, Yamamoto SS and Brosschot JF, 2010. The relationship of autonomic imbalance, heart rate variability and cardiovascular disease risk factors. *Int J Cardiol*. 141(2): 122–131.

Vickhoff B, Malmgren H, Aström R *et al.*, 2013. Music structure determines heart rate variability of singers. *Front Psychol*. 4: 334, 2013.

CHAPTER 4

Cervical and Thoracic Cardiac Branches

THE HEART AND EMOTIONS

INTRODUCTION

Our heart and emotions have a unique connection with each other and to the vagus nerve. The heart sends more signals through the vagus nerve to the brain than the brain sends to the heart. The signals from the heart significantly affect brain function, influencing emotional processing by the amygdala, as well as cognitive function. In this chapter, we will begin by describing the anatomy and physiology of the sympathetic and parasympathetic neural contributions to the cardiac plexus, the network of nerves supplying the heart. This will help us understand and appreciate the communication pathways between the heart and the brain and how they can be regulated, paying special attention to vagal function.

After discussing how vagal activity can be assessed by monitoring HRV, we will explore how emotions arise in the body from autonomic, visceral and muscular sensations and how these responses influence HRV. We will then describe how the HRV signal is further modified and processed by the limbic system and the prefrontal cortex to translate raw emotional sensations into conscious feelings. Finally, we will explore how emotions are encoded in the HRV and how those emotions that stimulate the vagus nerve improve physical, emotional and mental health, as illustrated in two case studies.

Some background

What is an emotion? According to the Merriam-Webster Dictionary, it is:

> A conscious mental reaction (such as anger or fear) subjectively experienced as strong feeling usually directed toward a specific object and typically accompanied by physiological and behavioral changes in the body.

The Oxford Reference Dictionary defines an emotion as:

> A state of arousal that can be experienced as pleasant or unpleasant. Emotions can have three components: for example, fear can involve an unpleasant subjective experience, an increase in physiological measures such as heart rate, and a tendency to flee from the situation provoking the fear.

Although definitions of emotion vary, they usually include a subjective experience, a distinct physiological pattern and a behavioral response. From a mechanistic perspective, emotions can be defined as "a positive or negative experience that is associated with a particular pattern of physiological activity" (Wikipedia 2023). Psychologist and author Dr Steven Pinker proposed that the original role of emotions was to motivate adaptive behaviors that in the past would have contributed to the passing on of genes through survival, reproduction and kin selection (Pinker 1997). Sometimes the words "emotion" and "feeling" are used interchangeably, but that is inaccurate. I would like to emphasize a fundamental difference between feelings and emotions: feelings are experienced consciously, whereas emotions manifest either consciously or subconsciously.

What part of your body responds the most vigorously to emotions? Probably most of you thought "heart." That is correct. We all recognize the sensation of a fast pounding in the chest as your heart responds to fear. But the heart does not just *respond* to emotions, it *creates* them. Emotions are formed by integration of all the signals that are coming from the brain and the body systems at a given moment. Where does that integration take place? Anatomy and physiology of the ANS indicates that it takes place in the heart. The heart then sends the integrated signal to the brain through the afferent nerve fibers in the sympathetic nerves and the vagus nerve in the form of the HRV. In this chapter, I will provide evidence that emotions are encoded in the HRV and that when the HRV signal reaches the amygdala, the code is read and identified. This information is passed on to the prefrontal cortex, or thinking part of the brain, and you become conscious of the emotion as a feeling.

For thousands of years, the heart has represented the center of emotions, spirituality and romance. As far back as the ancient Greeks, lyric poems that were written to be sung accompanied by music identified the heart with love. The lyrical poet Sappho, who lived during the 7th century BCE on the island of Lesbos surrounded by female disciples for whom she wrote passionate poems, agonized over her "mad heart" quaking with love. In "Ode to Aphrodite," she says:

> What is here the longing more than other
> Here in this mad heart?
> Come again to me! O now! Release me!
> End the great pang! And all my heart desireth
> Now of fulfilment, fulfil! O Aphrodite,
> Fight by my shoulder!

Among the ancient Romans, the link between the heart and love was commonplace. Romans worshipped a god called Cupid, who was the son of the goddess of love, Venus, and the god of war, Mars. He was depicted as a plump male infant, carrying a bow and arrow. The arrow could be one of two kinds: one with a sharp golden point, and the other with a blunt tip of lead. A person whose heart was wounded by the golden arrow was filled with uncontrollable desire, but the one whose heart was struck by the lead tip became revolted by the object of their affection and tried to flee.

The link between the heart and desire did not appear in northern Europe until the Middle Ages. One of the first known modern heart shapes appears in a detail from the French manuscript "The Romance of Alexander," dated 1344.

It is probable that the heart became associated with emotions early in history because people sensed changes in their heart when they felt deep emotions. The position of the heart in the center of the chest also means that sensations there have a very noticeable effect. Heartfelt experiences are so common that the link between the heart and emotions is embedded in our language. There are at least 40 or 50 idioms and expressions about the heart and the emotions it has come to symbolize, such as "breaking my heart," "change of heart," "with a heavy heart," "light-hearted humor," "pour your heart out," "have a heart-to-heart talk" and describing someone as "big-hearted."

In Sufi psychology, the heart refers to the spiritual heart or qalb, not the physical organ. It is this spiritual heart that contains the deeper intelligence and wisdom. Rumi, the Sufi poet, wrote:

The beauty of the heart
Is the lasting beauty;
Its lips give to drink
Of the water of life.
Truly it is the water,
That which pours,
And the one who drinks.
All three become one when
Your talisman is shattered.
That oneness you can't know
By reasoning.

(Mathnawi II, 716-718)

This is where the vagus nerve plays a role. In this chapter, I will present evidence that deliberately cultivating certain emotions, such as appreciation and gratitude, will stimulate the vagus nerve and bring you to a coherent autonomic state. Other studies show that being in the coherent state improves your cognitive skills and ability to regulate your emotions. In this way, vagal stimulation makes use of the heart-brain connection so you can access the "deeper intelligence and wisdom" referred to in the Sufi teachings.

ANATOMY AND PHYSIOLOGY OF THE CARDIAC PLEXUS

The network of nerves supplying the heart is called the cardiac plexus. It receives contributions from the right and left vagus nerves, as well as contributions from the sympathetic trunk. Approximately 50 percent of the sympathetic nerve fibers are afferent, and fifty percent are efferent. On the other hand, 80 percent of the parasympathetic nerve fibers are afferent, meaning that much more information is passing through the vagus nerve from the heart to the brain than from the brain to the heart. As will be demonstrated later in this chapter, the heart acts as a repository for sensory information coming from the rest of the body, which it then integrates and transmits to the limbic system of the brain. A simple diagram of the sympathetic and parasympathetic innervation of the heart is shown in Figure 4.1.

The black lines indicate the vagus nerve and left and right vagal cardiac branches that serve the heart, as well as the postganglionic vagal nerves at the sinoatrial (SA) node and the atrioventricular (AV) node. Stimulation of the efferent fibers of the vagal cardiac branches decreases heart rate by slowing down the cardiac pacemaker at the SA node and reducing atrial-ventricular conductance at the AV node. In this way, they can regulate blood pressure. The gray lines represent the pre- and postganglionic sympathetic nerves serving the heart and coronary arterioles. The sympathetic efferent nerves increase heart rate and myocardial contractility. They also cause contraction of veins, reducing venous blood volume capacity, and produce constriction of arterioles, leading to increased peripheral resistance and blood pressure.

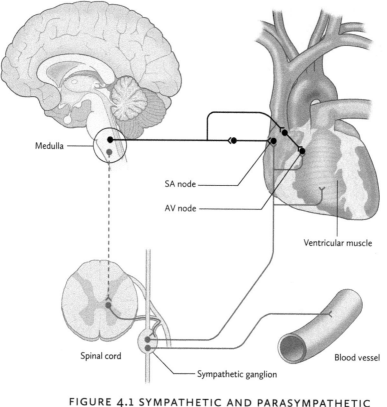

FIGURE 4.1 SYMPATHETIC AND PARASYMPATHETIC INNERVATION OF THE HEART.
SA node: sinoatrial node; AV node: atrioventricular node.
Source: Rocha et al. 2021, Figure 1.

Figure 4.1 illustrates that the heart is innervated with both sympathetic and para-sympathetic nerves and shows where the inputs are located. What is not clearly shown here is that the left and right cardiac vagal preganglionic nerves (black lines) also synapse onto parasympathetic ganglia, located in the epicardium (the connective tissue that envelops the heart) and in the atrial and ventricular septa (the cardiac tissue separating the left and right atria and ventricles) as described by Capilupi *et al.* (2020). These parasympathetic ganglionic neurons project postganglionic axons to different parts of the heart such as the walls of the left and right ventricles. When the efferent fibers of these neurons are stimulated, cardiac contractility is decreased so that the heart does not beat so forcefully.

Afferent fibers, located in the sympathetic and the parasympathetic cardiac nerves, pass sensory information (mechanical and chemical) from the heart to the brain. Cardiac sympathetic afferents are present in the atria and ventricles. Some are myelinated, meaning they are covered by an insulating myelin sheath, and some are unmyelinated. Myelination allows more rapid transmission of information along neural fibers from peripheral receptors to the central nervous system. Cardiac sympathetic afferent nerves work in conjunction with the arterial baroreceptors and cardiac vagal afferents to regulate cardiac function and maintain homeostasis. In pathological situations, they can also activate the cardiovascular system as a reflex response, leading to increases in blood pressure, heart rate and myocardial contractile function. For example, if the heart tissue is not receiving sufficient oxygen (myocardial ischemia), these sensory nerves will cause a sudden increase in heart rate (tachycardia) and transmit the sensation of pain (angina pectoris) to the brain.

Cardiac vagal afferent nerves innervate all chambers of the heart and can be divided into atrial myelinated fibers, ventricular myelinated fibers and cardiac receptors with unmyelinated fibers (Malliani *et al.* 1986). The atrial myelinated fibers respond to static and dynamic changes in the tension of the atrial walls caused by alterations in pressure and heart rate. Ventricular vagal receptors with myelinated fibers discharge in phase with the rise of the pressure in the ventricles. The responsiveness of the myelinated fibers to mechanical stimuli indicates they are primarily mechanosensitive in nature, although they can also be excited by various drugs. In general, atrial and ventricular unmyelinated fibers respond to pressure but they can also be markedly excited by chemical substances. They seem to mediate cardiovascular reflexes of a solely inhibitory nature, meaning that they act to reduce heart rate and blood pressure. A summary of the main functions of the cardiac nerves is shown in Table 4.1.

Table 4.1 Main functions of the cardiac nerves

Parasympathetic efferent fibers	**Vagal cardiac nerves** Function: reducing the heart rate, reducing the force of contraction of the heart, vasoconstriction of the coronary arteries

Sympathetic efferent fibers	**Cardiac nerves from the lower cervical and upper thoracic sympathetic ganglia** Function: increasing heart rate, increasing the force of contraction of the myocardium
Parasympathetic afferent fibers	**Vagal cardiac nerves** Function: feedback on blood pressure, bringing information from inner organs
Sympathetic afferent fibers	**Afferents to upper thoracic and lower cervical sympathetic ganglia** Function: feedback on blood pressure, pain sensation

To fully understand the importance of the afferent vagal innervation of the heart, it is necessary to appreciate that the chemical and mechanical changes in the heart to which these nerves respond arise not only from the heart itself but also from efferent sympathetic and parasympathetic nerve fibers from the brain and from the cardiac extrinsic ganglia in the thoracic cavity that are connected to the heart. These ganglia also connect directly to the lungs and esophagus and indirectly to other organs and structures, including skin and arteries, via the sympathetic chains on each side of the spinal cord. Armour (2008) has hypothesized that the heart has its own intrinsic nervous system, or "little brain," comprised of sensory (afferent), interconnecting (local) and motor (adrenergic and cholinergic efferent) neurons that communicate with those in the cardiac thoracic external ganglia, all under the influence of neural and hormonal inputs from the brain. The intrinsic cardiac neurons can also generate spontaneous activity independent of inputs from central and other intrathoracic neurons.

Based on experimental data cited in Armour (2008), it appears that the intrinsic cardiac afferent neurons transduce the local mechanical and chemical milieu of the heart to other neurons in their own cluster or ganglion, as well as to those in other intrinsic ganglia in different regions of the heart. In addition, they transmit the milieu data to the intrathoracic extracardiac ganglia that connect to the dorsal root ganglia in the spine. As a result, the heart's intrinsic nervous system transmits information to the brain via afferent neurons in the spine through the dorsal root ganglia as well as via the vagus nerve through the nodose ganglia and then to the nucleus solitarius, where the signals redirect to the limbic system and then to the prefrontal cortex. This model is illustrated in Figure 4.2.

There is a continual exchange of information within and between three circuits: (1) the intrinsic nervous system, (2) the extrinsic cardiac ganglia – dorsal root ganglia – spine circuit, and (3) the spine – medulla – limbic system – cortex circuit. The cardiac neuronal hierarchy is organized to provide the flexibility necessary for beat-to-beat coordination of cardiac functions on a regional basis via quick (intrinsic cardiac ganglia), medium (intrathoracic) and relatively slow feedback circuits (spinal cord and brain). Such information exchange among the neurons is also indirectly influenced by sensory inputs from receptors located in other body regions (Armour 1991). Hormonal, chemical and pressure information detected by receptors in the heart is translated into neurological impulses by the heart's intrinsic nervous system and is sent from the heart to the brain through the afferent pathways shown in Figure 4.2.

The resulting integrative signal that encompasses the continually changing chemical, hormonal and dynamic structural properties of the cardiac tissue is the HRV, how the heart rate changes with time. In this way, the heart functions not just as a pump but also as a repository of chemical and mechanical sensory signals arising in the heart, blood vessels, extracardiac ganglia and other organs, which it integrates into the HRV rhythmic information pattern it sends to the brain.

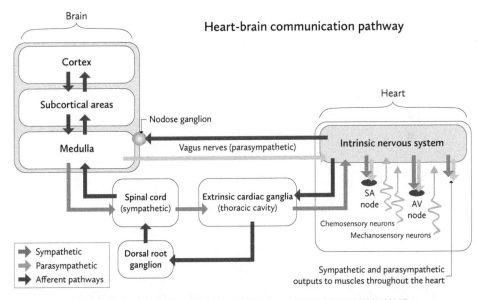

FIGURE 4.2 HEART-BRAIN COMMUNICATION PATHWAYS.
The neural communication pathways interacting between the heart and brain are responsible for the generation of HRV. The intrinsic cardiac nervous system integrates information from the extrinsic nervous system and the sensory neurites within the heart. The extrinsic cardiac ganglia located in the thoracic cavity have connections to the lungs and esophagus and are indirectly connected via the spinal cord to many other organs, including the skin and arteries. The vagus nerve (parasympathetic) primarily consists of afferent (flowing to the brain) fibers that connect to the medulla. The sympathetic afferent nerves first connect to the extrinsic cardiac ganglia (also a processing center), then to the dorsal root ganglion and the spinal cord. Once afferent signals reach the medulla, they travel to the subcortical areas (thalamus, amygdala, etc.) and then the higher cortical areas.
Source: © 2010 HeartMath Institute. www.heartmath.org.

HEART RATE VARIABILITY AS A MEASURE OF VAGAL ACTIVITY

Heart rate variability is defined as the fluctuation in the time interval between adjacent heartbeats as illustrated in Figure 4.3.

The electrocardiogram (ECG) is shown in gray on the bottom and the instantaneous heart rate is shown by the black line above. The time between each of the heartbeats (black line) between 0 and approximately 13 seconds becomes progressively shorter and heart rate accelerates and then starts to decelerate around 13 seconds. This pattern of heart rate accelerations and decelerations is the basis of the heart's rhythms.

This variation is generated by the interaction of the sympathetic and parasympathetic components of the ANS as they regulate heart rate, cardiac contractility, blood vessel diameter, blood pressure, gas exchange, gastrointestinal function, facial muscles and heart-brain interactions. Because the ANS regulates so many interdependent systems, heart rate oscillations are complex. This complexity in HRV provides the heart with the flexibility to rapidly cope with uncertain and changing inner internal and external environments. While healthy biological systems show spatial and temporal complexity, stressed systems involve a loss of complexity.

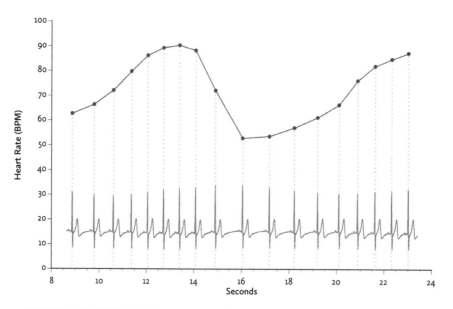

FIGURE 4.3 HEART RATE VARIABILITY WITH ELECTROCARDIOGRAM.
Source: © 2015 HeartMath Institute. www.heartmath.org.

Unless a person is suffering from a pathological cardiac condition, such as coronary artery disease or heart valve malfunction that produces an irregular heartbeat, a high resting HRV is favorable because it is associated with a strong ability to tolerate stress. In addition, higher levels of resting HRV are linked to superior performance of executive functions like attention and emotional processing by the prefrontal cortex (McCraty and Schaffer 2015). Since the vagus nerve is the main contributor to the parasympathetic component of the ANS, resting HRV can only reach high values if the vagus nerve is functioning optimally. Therefore, HRV is considered a measure of vagus function. Vagal activity is extremely important because poor function predicts death following a heart attack (Kleiger *et al.* 1987), cardiovascular reactivity to stressors (Muranaka *et al.* 1988) and heightened states of anxiety (Friedman and Thayer 1998).

So, what is a good value of HRV? One of the most common parameters used to quantify HRV is the standard deviation of inter-beat intervals (SDNN), as described in Chapter 2. Summary of data from 27 studies in which short-term (five-minute) measurements of HRV were taken in healthy participants revealed an average SDNN value of 50 ms (± 16 SD). Compared with men, women demonstrated slightly lower values for SDNN (45–46 ms) (Nunan *et al.* 2010). From these data, it seems prudent to aim for an SDNN value over 50 ms for short-term measurements. But HRV tends to decrease with age unless an effort is made to ensure that vagal function is optimized by using some of the techniques described in this book. So, what is a good value of HRV for your age? The results from a study involving 782 women and 1124 men (Voss *et al.* 2015), in which SDNN was measured for five minutes and the results grouped according to gender and age, are shown in Table 4.2.

Table 4.2 Effect of chronological age on heart rate variability

Age (yrs)	25–34	35–44	45–54	55–64	65–74
SDNN (women)	48.7 ± 19.0	45.4 ± 20.5	36.9 ± 13.8	30.6 ± 12.4	27.8 ± 11.8
SDNN (men)	50.0 ± 20.9	44.6 ± 16.8	36.8 ± 14.6	32.8 ± 14.7	29.6 ± 13.2

Even though these data show a sharp decline in SDNN with age, it does not have to be like that. I just measured my SDNN for five minutes using a portable monitor connected to some free "HRV Logger" software. My SDNN was 62.5 ms. I will be 68 years old in two weeks. Regardless of the published averages, a good value for your SDNN if you are middle-aged or older is over 50 ms. If you are in your 20s, based on my experience teaching undergraduate students to measure their own HRV, I would say aim for 75 ms or higher.

When you are reviewing measurements of HRV, it is essential to take note of whether the participants in the study were breathing normally or were deliberately breathing more deeply and slowly than usual. All the data we have discussed so far were measured while the participants were breathing normally. This is important because if you breathe at about six breaths per minute instead of the more usual 12–15 breaths per minute, your HRV will be higher than your normal reading due to the enhanced contribution to HRV of respiratory sinus arrhythmia (RSA), as explained in Chapter 2. (A mechanistic explanation of how breathing more deeply and slowly than normal stimulates the vagus nerve and increases HRV will be provided in Chapter 5.) Daily practice of this technique leads to deep, slow breathing without any conscious effort, and this becomes your new "normal" way of breathing. People with this skill will show an enhanced RSA contribution to their HRV when they breathe at their usual rate (now about six breaths per minute), and their SDNN will be significantly higher than average for their age cohort.

As described in Chapter 2, RMSSD is another common parameter used to quantify HRV. This parameter just reflects the parasympathetic component of HRV because it only includes very fast beat-to-beat changes in HRV, instead of the more gradual changes that take several heartbeats or longer to establish themselves. Just as a reminder, the parasympathetic, or vagal, response is mediated by release of the neurotransmitter acetylcholine, which acts very quickly compared to the sympathetic neurotransmitter norepinephrine. For this reason, the vagal response is manifested in the heart by quick beat-to-beat changes in HRV. Healthy values of RMSSD are similar in value to those described for SDNN.

HOW EMOTIONS ARE FELT IN THE BODY

Emotional experience is the combination of stimuli the brain receives from external environment and the internal sensations transmitted to the brain from bodily organs and systems. The stimuli from the environment are received directly by the sensory organs of the head and neck in the form of sight, hearing, touch, smell and taste. There is no need for these messages to be transmitted along the spinal cord. You feel emotions in your body at three levels: autonomic, visceral and muscular, or somatic. For example, after I meditate, the emotion I feel is satisfaction. Most of the stimuli I am sensing are internal rather than from the external environment because I meditate in a quiet place. On an autonomic level, my heart rate is low. I can barely feel it beating because the contractility is small.

What about on a visceral level? The word visceral has two meanings, the first relating to the soft internal organs of the body, including the lungs, the heart and the organs of the digestive, excretory, reproductive and circulatory systems, and the second to deep, inward feelings rather than intellectual thoughts. On a visceral level, my heart feels soft, my digestive organs settled, and inwardly I feel calm and peaceful. On a somatic level, my forehead, jaw and tongue feel relaxed, and my lips, cheeks and fingers feel plump and full. The lips are innervated with parasympathetic nerves (Izumi *et al.* 2006) that dilate the blood vessels and increase circulation, making the lips feel plump. Just run your fingers lightly over your lips to stimulate these vagal nerve endings. It is an easy way to relax. All the sensations I experience after meditation are telling me that my vagus nerve is fully engaged. The emotion of satisfaction is good for my body.

An example of an emotion that causes severe damage to the body is broken-heart syndrome. Broken-heart syndrome occurs when a patient experiences severe emotional distress that they literally feel in their heart. Their hormones surge and the heart's left ventricle swells, adopting a rounded shape with a narrow neck like a takotsubo (a Japanese octopus trap, Figure 4.4), hence the syndrome's official name, which causes it to pump blood less efficiently.

Nasser Khan, a cardiologist who is Medical Director of the Structural Heart Program at Methodist Health System, describes the syndrome as follows: "The apex of the heart really bulges and doesn't move, and patients present with acute chest pain, shortness of breath, kind of like a heart attack, but when you do an angiogram, you find their heart arteries are fine, no blockages" (Golembiewski 2021). In his practice, Khan says that he sees patients with broken-heart syndrome once or twice a month. When considering the mind-body connection, Khan says: "they're unbelievably interconnected, the mind and body go hand in hand."

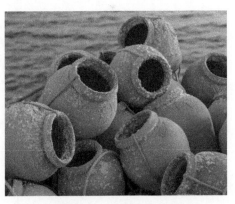

FIGURE 4.4 TRADITIONAL JAPANESE OCTOPUS TRAPS.

HOW EMOTIONS ARE GENERATED – A QUICK GUIDE TO THE LIMBIC SYSTEM

As described previously and illustrated in Figure 4.2, HRV is a dynamic signal that is continually being modified by mechanical and chemical information coming from the intrinsic nervous system of the heart, and from the other visceral organs via the extrinsic cardiac ganglia and the spinal cord. This sensory information, which contributes to the emotional experience, is transmitted to the nucleus solitarius in the medulla via visceral sensory (afferent) nerve fibers in the sympathetic chain adjacent to the spinal cord and by those in the vagus nerve.

Once the afferent signals reach the medulla, they travel to the limbic system. The HRV signal is modified by information coming to the limbic system from the five senses via special visceral and somatic afferent nerves, and by signals sent from the skeletal muscles via somatic sensory nerves. The sum of all these inputs into the HRV signal forms the basis of the emotional state. As will be explained in the next section, each emotion is characterized by a specific combination of autonomic, visceral and somatic sensory signals that is encoded in the time and frequency domain aspects of the HRV. Figure 4.5 illustrates the processes involved in emotional sensing.

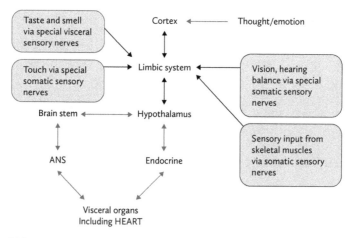

FIGURE 4.5 PHYSIOLOGY OF MIND-BODY INTERACTION.

The limbic system is important because it mediates communication between the mind and the body. Regarding the emotions, the most relevant part of the limbic system is the amygdala. Figure 4.6 illustrates the connections between the different components of the limbic system.

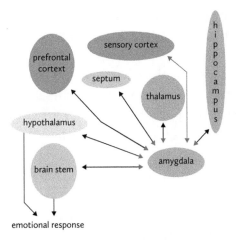

FIGURE 4.6 COMPONENTS OF THE LIMBIC SYSTEM.
Source: Used by permission of "The Brain from Top to Bottom." Topic: "Emotions and the Brain." https://thebrain.mcgill.ca/flash/i/i_04/i_04_cr/i_04_cr_peu/i_04_cr_peu.html.

Notice all the bi-directional connections between the amygdala, the brain stem, the cortical features and the additional components of the limbic system (thalamus, hypothalamus, amygdala and hippocampus). The septum is sometimes considered a part of the limbic system because it is connected to other limbic structures. It is involved in processing rewarding experiences and has other roles about which little is known in humans. Thalamus is Greek for "inner room" and it is known as the "gateway to the brain." Nearly all sensory inputs from the outside and from the inner body pass through it to the cerebral cortex.

The hypothalamus sits under the thalamus at the top of brain stem. Although small, it controls many critical bodily functions including the ANS and the endocrine system, as well as temperature regulation, food intake, water balance and sleep-wake cycles. The amygdala is a limbic structure that is essential for decoding emotions and for warning the body about certain stimuli that might threaten its survival. As a result of evolution, many of the body's alarm circuits are grouped together in the amygdala. Consequently, many sensory inputs converge in the amygdala to inform it of potential dangers in its environment. The amygdala also receives numerous connections from the hippocampus, which is involved in storing and retrieving explicit memories. This may be the reason that memories connected with an important emotional event are etched deeply into our consciousness.

The HRV signal travels from the heart to the nucleus solitarius in the brain stem to the amygdala. As seen in Figure 4.6, the amygdala also receives input from the sensory cortex in the brain relating to the five senses that further modifies the HRV signal. The HRV signal that is received by the amygdala, after incorporating the additional sensory data and possibly signals related to relevant memories from the hippocampus, is a record of the emotional state at that moment. Perhaps it looks like the HRV signal shown in Figure 4.7.

Karl Pribram, a neurosurgeon and scientific researcher, developed a theory of emotion in which he proposed that past experiences (inside and outside the body) set up familiar patterns in neural architecture, such as HRV (Pribram and Melges 1969). These stable patterns help organize feelings and perceptions by creating a set of "expectancies" against which incoming signals from physiological behaviors, such as breathing, eating and sleeping, are compared. New input patterns are compared to the old ones and mismatches are detected. Mismatches generate new emotions.

The amygdala is continually receiving signals from all over the body and it processes each type of signal, such as HRV, by comparing it to the existing stable patterns it has set up from past experiences and contexts. Data are extracted from the HRV signal associated with the level of arousal (high or low) and the valence of the experience (positive or negative). As will be shown later, this information appears to be encoded in the frequency spectrum of the HRV. A signal reflecting high arousal and negative valence could mean a person is experiencing fear, and the amygdala would have to alert the body to adopt survival mode and behave accordingly.

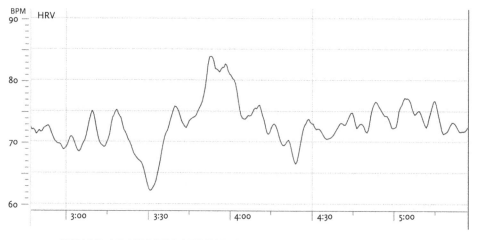

FIGURE 4.7 HEART RATE VARIABILITY OF A PERSON AT REST.
Heart rate is in beats per minute, time is in minutes and seconds.

On the other hand, a signal reflecting low to medium arousal and a single frequency peak centered around 0.1 Hz (6 cycles per minute), as illustrated in

Figure 4.8, would indicate that the person is in a state of sympathetic/parasympathetic balance associated with a feeling of relaxed alertness.

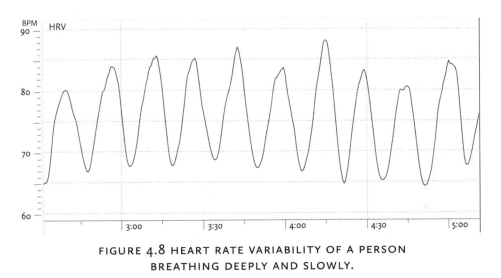

FIGURE 4.8 HEART RATE VARIABILITY OF A PERSON
BREATHING DEEPLY AND SLOWLY.

When the HRV signal reaches the prefrontal cortex, or "thinking part of the brain" that is responsible for reasoning, decision making, problem solving, comprehension and impulse control, you become aware of your emotional experience as a feeling, such as fear, anger, joy or satisfaction. At this point, the signal can be modified with conscious intention. You can decide to tone down your anger by taking a deep breath and releasing the tension in your jaw. The modified signal is sent back to the intrinsic nervous system of the heart and other organs via the ANS, resulting in changes in physiological function. For further information on theories of emotion, I highly recommend an article by McCraty (2015), "Heart brain neurodynamics. The making of emotions."

EMOTIONS THAT STIMULATE THE VAGUS NERVE

Results suggest that positive emotions, such as appreciation and gratitude, lead to changes in HRV, which may be beneficial in the treatment of hypertension and in reducing the likelihood of sudden death in patients with congestive heart failure and coronary artery disease. McCraty et al. (1995) assessed HRV in 24 healthy participants for a five-minute baseline period and again when they were asked to experience either appreciation or anger using a mental exercise for which they had previously received training.

Briefly, half of the participants were instructed to consciously disengage from unpleasant mental and emotional reactions by shifting their attention to the heart and to focus on sincerely feeling appreciation toward someone, or something, in their life. The other participants were asked to self-induce the emotion of anger by recalling situations in their lives that still caused feelings of anger and/or frustration. This self-recall method has been shown to effectively induce the emotional states of anger and frustration.

All participants were asked to maintain the desired feelings for five minutes, which was the maximal time that most subjects could sustain the emotional focus. Comparison of the time-domain recordings (heart rate versus time) revealed that most subjects developed a rhythmic sine wave-like pattern during appreciation, similar to the HRV pattern shown during the coherent state, but this pattern was not seen for baseline recordings, or for anger. Figure 4.9A shows an HRV recording of one of my students watching a live horse while sending the horse a feeling of appreciation. Heart rate was recorded for three minutes. The characteristic wave-like appearance of the coherent state is evident.

Figure 4.9B shows a frequency domain analysis of the same data. A fast Fourier transform (FFT) converts a signal from the time domain (signal strength as a function of time) to the frequency domain (signal strength as a function of frequency). Signal strength is expressed in terms of "power spectral density" and is associated with the height of the peak. The Fourier transform shows the signal's spectral content, as a function of frequency (Hz). This type of analysis gives us information about the *pattern* with which heart rate varies with time, or, more precisely, the frequencies of oscillation of HRV.

Looking at Figure 4.9B, you can see that the peak oscillation frequency is close to 0.1 Hz, or six cycles per minute. That frequency is within the narrow band of frequencies associated with coherence, where the sympathetic and parasympathetic components of ANS are closely interacting in time with the breath. The frequency spectra of baseline recordings are usually much less organized and consist of many low-amplitude peaks scattered over a wide range of frequencies. In simple terms, peaks at lower frequencies imply that there is a sympathetic predominance, and peaks at higher frequencies, a parasympathetic predominance. Sometimes there will be simultaneous peaks at both frequency ranges, indicating the presence of sympathetic and parasympathetic activity but opposing each other rather than working together.

In the 1995 study by McCraty *et al.*, both anger and appreciation caused an overall increase in autonomic activation as indicated by amplitude of HRV and the total power of the FFT over the recorded frequency range. The two emotional states, however, could be distinguished by their power spectral analyses. Although both emotional states produced an increase in sympathetic activity, in the case of anger there was very little parasympathetic, or vagal, contribution.

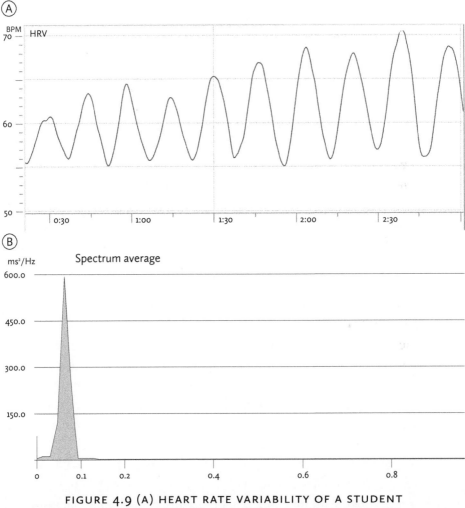

FIGURE 4.9 (A) HEART RATE VARIABILITY OF A STUDENT WATCHING A HORSE (TIME DOMAIN WITH TIME IN MINUTES AND SECONDS). (B) FREQUENCY DOMAIN OF THE SAME DATA.

Emerging research indicates that HRV is significantly associated with higher blood flow in the prefrontal cortex and the amygdala (Thayer *et al.* 2012) and with greater connectivity between the prefrontal cortex and the amygdala (Sakaki *et al.* 2016). This pattern is associated with improved skill at regulating emotions (Etkin *et al.* 2015). By scanning the felt sensations in your body, you can tune into emotions before you become conscious of them. If it is a negative emotion you are feeling, these sensations can be detrimental to the body – for example, digestion can be impaired. By becoming aware of these sensations at an early stage, you have an opportunity to modify your stress response and stop the damage that trauma is causing in your body. This approach is termed "somatic experiencing" and will be discussed in Chapter 7.

CASE STUDY: Shifting to calm with heartfelt gratitude
Ann L. Baldwin, PhD, Physiologist, HeartMath Certified Trainer, Usui Reiki Master, Mind-Body-Science (abaldwin@mind-body-science.com)

KC came to me in my office for biofeedback to address problems with anxiety. She was in her early 50s, happily married with children, and was a senior engineering manager in an innovative technologies company. Her job was challenging, but she had been well able to cope with stressful situations for many years and enjoyed solving the complex problems that she faced on a day-to-day basis. However, a year or so ago she started to suffer from anxiety which was adversely affecting her ability as a public speaker. She was familiar with biofeedback from her past and decided to give it a try.

When she came in for her first session, I noticed that she was well turned-out and organized. She was very respectful of my credentials, spoke clearly and came straight to the point. As a top-level manager, she knew that time was of the essence both for her and for me. She said that her most pressing problem was the anxiety that overtook her when she got up to speak in public. Words would escape her, and her mind would go blank. She emphasized that this was not how it used to be.

I started by taking a baseline recording of her heart rate variability (HRV) (Figure 4.10A). Her average heart rate was 82.4 bpm, a little high, and her heart rate varied with time in a random pattern, sometimes increasing and sometimes decreasing with no apparent pattern. This type of HRV signal is very common and indicates an imbalance of the autonomic nervous system. Heart rate variability reflects the ability of the heart to adapt to the body's needs (including the brain), and the higher its value, the better the heart can minutely control blood flow according to the needs of the various organs and muscles. Her baseline HRV was 37 ms, which is low – I like to see values above 50 ms for people in their 50s. Likewise, her vagus nerve was functioning at a low level, 34 ms instead of 50 ms or higher. Her coherence, or balance between sympathetic and parasympathetic function, was also low, at 34%. When a person is experiencing good autonomic balance, they can reach a coherence of 100%. These readings indicated that KC was operating in "fight or flight" mode, rather than "rest and digest," which made her a prime candidate for learning heartfelt gratitude.

To begin with, I taught her the HeartMath technique, Heart-Focused Breathing™ (HFB), in which one focuses on one's heart or chest area; as one breathes, one imagines the breath entering and leaving one's heart, while breathing slightly more deeply and slowly than usual. I also asked her to consciously relax all her muscles on every exhale. After a few moments, I asked her how she felt, and she answered, "Calm in my body." She repeated the exercise, and this time I recorded her HRV. The result is shown in Figure 4.10B. Now the HRV pattern was rhythmic rather than random, each pulse lasting about nine seconds. This meant that her breathing and HRV were synchronized, her heart rate increasing with each inhale and decreasing with each exhale, indicating a high level of coherence. The data reflected this new state; her HRV was 66 ms, vagus function was 61 ms and coherence 70 percent. She had experienced a shift to vagus stimulation and her autonomic nervous system was in much better balance. I asked her to practice HFB twice a day during the week before her next session when I planned to introduce an exercise in gratitude.

During the next session, I introduced her to the HeartMath technique Quick Coherence™ (QC) which starts with HFB and then the client is asked to breathe in a "heart feeling." That means that they imagine a simple experience that brings them warm feelings of genuine appreciation and gratitude in their heart. It could be feeling the emotions or sensations associated with stroking a pet, lying on the beach or seeing the face of a loved one. KC chose to feel gratitude for the beautiful layers of clouds she sees from the window of the plane when she is traveling for work. When I asked her how she felt, she said it "opened up her heart."

During the next week, she practiced HFB and QC. At our next session, she mentioned that she had used HFB successfully to rebalance herself and relax her tight chest after an aggressive phone call. She also said that when she practiced QC, she felt her stomach gurgling. This is a sign that the vagus nerve is being stimulated to wake up the digestion. When we did QC together at our session, she had some difficulty with distracting thoughts that prevented her from tuning into heart feelings of gratitude. I suggested that she try to regain some of the former happiness in her life that she had lost.

During the following week, KC spent time with her family on vacation and experienced some happy moments that she stored in her memory and enjoyed recalling. When we practiced QC together, she relived how she felt when she watched her daughter's glowing, happy face. After she finished, she said, "I need more of that!"

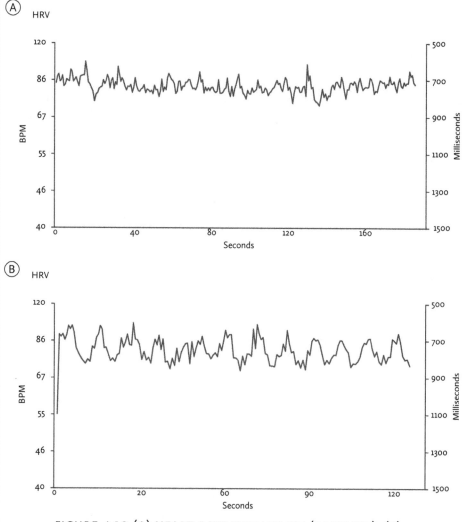

FIGURE 4.10 (A) HEART RATE VARIABILITY (BASELINE). (B) HEART RATE VARIABILITY (HEART-FOCUSED BREATHING).

One week later, KC had her last session with me before embarking on a period of work-related travel. KC was late for the session due to unexpected traffic conditions and was pleased to report that this problem did not cause her anxiety, as it would have done prior to her biofeedback training with me. We did QC together and she brought in a heartfelt feeling of gratitude by picturing her daughter's joyful face. I recorded her HRV, and even though she felt a little "test anxiety" because I was recording, her HRV was high at 61 ms, and her vagus function was 70 ms, which was the highest I had ever recorded from her.

In our conversation, KC indicated that she was now experiencing increased self-compassion, was able to be gentler with herself and had access to more ideas when giving advice to others. She was looking forward to a busier time at work after her well-earned time for self-reflection.

> Gratitude is one of the most powerful human emotions. Once expressed, it changes attitude, brightens outlook, and broadens our perspective. (Germany Kent)

CASE STUDY: Appreciating nature brings simultaneous calm and focus
Ann L. Baldwin, PhD, Physiologist, HeartMath Certified Trainer, Usui Reiki Master, Mind-Body-Science (abaldwin@mind-body-science.com)

ES had been seeing me for a year or so for Reiki and biofeedback to enhance his creativity as a writer and to calm his stomach. Through me, he became interested in horses and he even owned a horse for a while. In my practice, Mind-Body-Science, I encourage clients to enhance their experience of practicing biofeedback by interacting with horses who are specially selected and trained for this work. As prey animals, horses are sensitive to subtle changes in the environment, such as a person walking towards them, and they respond by showing body language such as ear movements, head turns and posture shifts. These can range from looking curiously at the person to walking towards them or turning away, depending largely on the person's level of arousal and emotional state. In this way, horses provide instant biofeedback, making them excellent partners in improving one's communication skills and self-awareness. ES enjoyed coming to visit the horses at the ranch because they made him feel calm and often provided him with personal insights that were useful in his work as an author.

One day, ES came to visit my horse, Major, at the ranch. Major was turned out loose in a large arena. ES greeted him, opened the gate and walked in with me, as usual. This time I noticed straight away that ES was uneasy. He seemed distracted, speaking briefly about various topics that did not seem to relate to each other, and not really taking much notice of the horse. Major, nose down, searched for shreds of hay on the ground and did not show any interest in ES. At this point, I realized that ES needed something extra, and I decided it might be better to continue the session outside the arena among the surrounding natural desert vegetation. I suggested that ES take Major for a relaxing walk to a nearby small, dry riverbed, known as a "wash." I secured a halter around Major's head and gave ES the attached rope so he could lead Major to the wash. As he was leading the horse, I instructed him to breathe a little more slowly and deeply than usual.

Breathing slower than normal, at about six breaths per minute (five seconds in, five seconds out), synchronizes respiration with heart rate variability, so that each exhale is accompanied by a shift from sympathetic to parasympathetic stimulation, producing a noticeable reduction in heart rate. With a long exhale, less blood is returned from the veins to the heart, and, consequently, less blood is pumped by the heart into the arteries. This means that the heart chambers and main artery are temporarily less stretched, and the sensory receptors in their walls reduce the stimulation of the nearby sympathetic nerve endings. This response allows the ventral vagus nerve fibers in the cardiac nerve branch to take over and shift the autonomic nervous system from to "fight or flight" to "rest and digest."

As ES walked along the road, I could see that his walking rhythm had naturally synchronized with that of the horse. Major's front hooves were hitting the ground exactly in time with the soles of ES's feet. This phenomenon, sometimes termed "entrainment," is often observed when two people walk together side by side; its frequency is far above what might be expected by chance. An example of unconscious synchronized walking is shown in Figure 4.11.

At present, it is not known what sensory mechanisms are employed to synchronize the walking patterns, but it happens more frequently if there is tactile contact between the two people. In this case, the lead rope was linking the horse to ES.

When ES entered the wash, he commented on how nice it was to be in nature and he noticed for the first time the fragrance of the

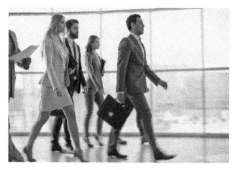

FIGURE 4.11 EXAMPLE OF TWO PEOPLE WALKING IN SYNCHRONY.

plants after a recent rainfall. ES commented on a pair of native Arizona birds, roadrunners, at the edge of the wash and pointed out how the male was fluffing up his feathers to attract the female. It was interesting to see how quickly he had shifted from a low-energy, somewhat scattered emotional condition, to a state of relaxed alertness, appreciating and taking interest in what was happening in the present moment while remaining calm and at ease. Published research shows that walking in green areas, near trees and water, for 15–30 minutes twice a week, reduces stress hormones, improves vitality and staves off depression (Hunter *et al.* 2019). At times, Major would stop walking for a few minutes, giving ES more chance to appreciate the natural environment and slip into "horse-time." ES said that Major was calming him. His heart felt expanded and he felt more than just an individual.

After we returned to the ranch, I introduced ES to another horse he had not met before. That horse imme-diately took notice of ES, who was now in a more approachable state, and continued to pay him attention. This seemed to boost ES's confi-dence and well-being. ES was so happy that he asked if he could take a photo of Major and me. The photo (Figure 4.12) shows the gen-tle, dreamy state we both entered during the walk with ES.

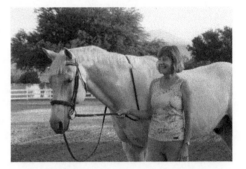

FIGURE 4.12 ANN AND MAJOR AFTER NATURE WALK.

Practicing heart focused breathing while walking in nature puts one in a relaxed but alert state so one can absorb more information from the environment. The trees smell more fragrant, the colors are brighter, one starts to notice the birds singing. Not only that – it helps shift people toward a state of deep relaxation and parasympathetic activity, which improves digestion and immune function and activates parts of the brain that help regulate emotions, leading to enhanced relationships (Song *et al.* 2015).

REFERENCES

Armour JA, 1991. Intrinsic cardiac neurons. *Journal Cardiovasc Electrophyiol.* 2: 331–341.
Armour JA, 2008. Potential clinical relevance of the "little brain" on the mammalian heart. *Experimental Physiology.* 93(2): 165–176. doi: 10.1113/expphysiol.2007.041178.

Capilupi MJ, Kerath SM and Becker LB, 2020. Vagus nerve stimulation and the cardiovascular system. *Cold Spring Harb Perspect Med*. 2020. doi: 10.1101/cshperspect.a034173.

Etkin A, Büchel C and Gross JJ, 2015. The neural bases of emotion regulation. *Nature Reviews Neuroscience*. 16(11): 693.

Friedman BH and Thayer JF, 1998. Anxiety and autonomic flexibility: a cardiovascular approach. *Biological Psychology*. 47(3): 243–263.

Golembiewski K, 2021. How the heart became the symbol of love, lust and the soul. Available from: www.discovermagazine.com/health/how-the-heart-became-the-symbol-of-love-lust-and-the-soul.

Hunter RF, Cleland C, Cleary A *et al.*, 2019. Environmental, health, wellbeing, social and equity effects of urban green space interventions: a meta-narrative evidence synthesis. *Environ Int*. 130: 104923. doi: 10.1016/j.envint.2019.104923.

Izumi H, Ishii H and Niioka T, 2006. Parasympathetic vasodilator fibers in the orofacial region. *Journal of Oral Biosciences*. 48(1): 30–41. doi: 10.1016/S1349-0079(06)80017-4.

Kleiger RE, Miller JP, Bigger JT Jr and Moss AJ, 1987. Decreased heart rate variability and its association with increased mortality after acute myocardial infarction. *Am J Cardiol*. 59(4): 256–262. doi: 10.1016/0002-9149(87)90795-8.

Malliani A, Lombardi F and Pagani M, 1986. Sensory innervation of the heart. In Cervero F and Morrison JFB (Eds). *Progress in Brain Research*. Vol. 67. Elsevier Science Publishers B.V.

McCraty R, Atkinson M, Tiller WA *et al.*, 1995. The effects of emotions on short-term power spectrum analysis of heart rate variability. *Am J Cardiol*. 76(14): 1089–1093. doi: 10.1016/s0002-9149(99)80309-9. Erratum in: *Am J Cardiol*. 1996 Feb 1; 77(4): 330.

McCraty R and Shaffer F, 2015. Heart rate variability: new perspectives on physiological mechanisms, assessment of self-regulatory capacity, and health risk. *Glob Adv Health Med*. 4: 46–61. doi: 10.7453/gahmj.2014.073.

McCraty R, 2015. Heart-brain neurodynamics. The making of emotions. In: Dahlitz M and Hall G (Eds). *Issues of the Heart: The Neuropsychotherapist*. Brisbane: Dahlitz Media; pp. 76–110.

Muranaka M, Lane JD, Suarez EC *et al.*, 1988. Stimulus-specific patterns of cardiovascular reactivity in Type A and B subjects: evidence for enhanced vagal reactivity in Type B. *Psychophysiology*. 25: 330–338.

Nunan D, Sandercock GR and Brodie DA, 2010. A quantitative systematic review of normal values for short-term heart rate variability in healthy adults. *Pacing Clin Electrophysiol*. 33(11): 1407–1417. doi: 10.1111/j.1540-8159.2010.02841-x.

Pinker S, 1997. *How the Mind Works*. New York: W.W. Norton & Company; p. 342.

Pribram KH and Melges FT, 1969. Psychophysiological basis of emotion. In: Vinken PJ and Bruyn GW (Eds). *Handbook of Clinical Neurology*. Amsterdam: North-Holland Publishing Company; pp. 316–341.

Rocha EA, Mehta N, Tavora-Mehta MZP *et al.*, 2021. Dysautonomia: a forgotten condition. Part 1. *Arquivos Brasileiros de Cardiologia*. 116(4): 814–835. doi: 10.36660/abc.20200420.

Sakaki M, Yoo HJ, Nga L *et al.*, 2016. Heart rate variability is associated with amygdala functional connectivity with MPFC across younger and older adults. *Neuroimage*. 139: 44–52.

Song C, Ikei H, Kobayashi M *et al.*, 2015. Effect of forest walking on autonomic nervous system activity in middle-aged hypertensive individuals: a pilot study. *Int J Environ Res Public Health*. 12: 2687–2699. doi: 10.3390/ijerph120302687.

Thayer JF, Åhs F, Fredrikson M *et al.*, 2012. A meta-analysis of heart rate variability and neuroimaging studies: implications for heart rate variability as a marker of stress and health. *Neuroscience and Biobehavioral Reviews*. 36(2): 747–756.

Voss A, Schroeder R, Heitmann A *et al.*, 2015. Short-term heart rate variability: influence of gender and age in healthy subjects. *PLoS One*. 10(3): e0118308. doi: 10.1371/journal.pone.0118308.

Wikipedia 2023. Emotion. Available from: https://en.wikipedia.org/wiki/Emotion.

CHAPTER 5

Pulmonary Branches

BREATH CONTROL AND LAUGHTER

INTRODUCTION

Many people have no idea that the way you breathe affects your sympathetic/ parasympathetic balance, your stress level and, hence, your HRV. The Reverend Stephen Hales (1733) was the first to notice that pulse rate varied with respiration, and in 1847, Carl Ludwig was the first to record the contribution that respiration makes to HRV, known as respiratory sinus arrhythmia (RSA). In this chapter, we provide a possible mechanistic explanation of how breathing more deeply and slowly than normal maximizes the activity of the vagus nerve and increases HRV. It should be noted that there is still some controversy about the relative importance of the different factors thought to contribute to HRV and the role played by the sympathetic nerves in manifesting RSA.

Next, we will describe the physiological benefits of increasing RSA and provide two breathing exercises to achieve this goal. This will be followed by accounts of two personal experiences that demonstrate how breathing more slowly and deeply than usual can improve inner clarity and banish frustration. Finally, we will present laughter yoga as another way to activate the vagus nerve by utilizing the forced exhale produced by laughter, and illustrate it with a case study.

RESPIRATORY CONTRIBUTION TO HRV

As described in Chapter 3, the vagus nerve is influenced by voluntary and involuntary cycles of respiration. Voluntary changes in respiration occur when you choose to sing or laugh. When you inhale, the vagal activity is reduced and so your heart beats faster, but as you exhale, the vagus nerve is more fully engaged and your heart beats more slowly. This effect, known as respiratory sinus arrhythmia (RSA), is maximized if you breathe more deeply and slowly than usual. *This is the easiest way to increase your HRV.* A simultaneous recording of chest expansion during respiration and HRV of a high-school student for 90 seconds is shown in Figure 5.1. There are two factors of note. One is that the student's HRV is perfectly synchronized with her respiration rate, each maximal value of heart rate coinciding with the associated maximal chest expansion. The student is in a state of coherence, and she is breathing at 6.5 breaths per minute. The second factor of note is the high amplitude of the HRV signal, with her heart rate ranging from 60–90 bpm in one breath. The high degree of HRV is a sign of youth and, when combined with a state of coherence, of a well-regulated ANS.

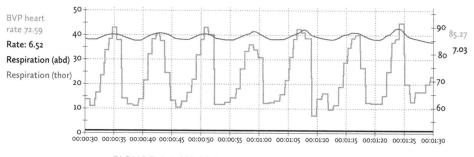
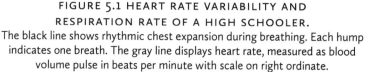

FIGURE 5.1 HEART RATE VARIABILITY AND
RESPIRATION RATE OF A HIGH SCHOOLER.
The black line shows rhythmic chest expansion during breathing. Each hump indicates one breath. The gray line displays heart rate, measured as blood volume pulse in beats per minute with scale on right ordinate.

What is special about breathing at six breaths per minute?

Why does breathing at about 5–7 breaths per minute synchronize respiration with HRV and maximize the amplitude of HRV? One explanation is that there are two physiological rhythms that strongly influence heart rate and can be coordinated to produce high-amplitude heart rate oscillations. The first rhythm is mediated by the baroreflex response. Baroreceptors are receptors located in the aortic arch and carotid arteries that are sensitive to blood pressure (BP). When the BP momentarily increases and the blood vessels are stretched, the baroreceptors signal to the nucleus solitarius in the brain stem to direct the heart, through the limbic system, to slow down. This takes 4–6.5 seconds. The slowing of the heart means that not so much blood is being pumped into these arteries and the BP decreases. As a result, the baroreceptors relax and respond by sending a message to the brain to speed up the heart to increase BP.

These back-and-forth responses create oscillations in heart rate and BP, such that each one lasts twice as long as the communication delay between brain and heart (4–6.5 seconds to slow down the heart and another 4–6.5 seconds to speed it up again, giving 8–13 seconds per oscillation). This means that there are 4.5–7.5 oscillations per minute (60 seconds divided by number of seconds per oscillation), or 0.075– 0.125 oscillations per second (Hz). As a result, there is a natural BP oscillation which has a frequency of about 0.1 Hz. This rhythm, known as "Mayer waves," was first noticed in 1833. The origin is uncertain, but they are thought to be a combination of sympathetic variation in regulation of blood vessel diameter and sympathetic and parasympathetic variation in control of heart rate.

The second major influence over HRV is respiration. As shown in Figure 5.1, as we inhale, the heart rate tends to increase, and as we exhale, the heart rate tends to decrease. Most people usually breathe at a faster frequency (i.e., between 0.15 and 0.4 Hz, or 9–24 breaths per minute) than that of the baroreflex response (4.5–7.5 breaths per minute). However, unlike the baroreflex response, which we cannot change, we *can* alter the pace of our own breathing. When breathing is slowed down to the same frequency as the baroreflex response, about 5–7 breaths per minute, this creates resonance. Both physiological rhythms vibrate in phase with each other and reinforce each other, greatly increasing the amplitude of the HRV oscillation. Thus, at an individual's resonance frequency, there is the potential for high-amplitude oscillations in HRV (Song and Lehrer 2003; Lehrer and Gevirtz 2014). An excellent way to demonstrate the concept of resonance is by using Barton's pendulums (Figure 5.2).

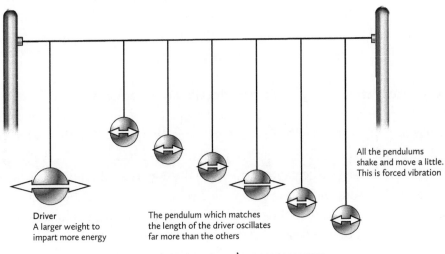

FIGURE 5.2 BARTON'S PENDULUMS.
Source: www.fizzics.org.

The heavier weight on the left is the driver which imparts energy to all the other pendulums. When it is moved, all the other weights will oscillate or sway a little but the pendulum which exactly matches the length of the driver will oscillate far more than all the others. That is resonance.

HOW DOES THE VAGUS NERVE MAXIMIZE RSA?

The answer to this question is two-fold. First, the vagus nerve is vital in regulating heart rate, and, second, its activity is highly influenced by inhalation and exhalation. The primary pacemaker of the heart is the sinoatrial node positioned in the right atrium and has a natural frequency of about 90 beats per minute (Sukhova and Mazurov 2007) which is above normal resting heart rate. The node is regulated by the ANS. The sympathetic nervous system and the vagus nerve transmit impulses from a cardiopulmonary oscillator consisting of neurons that connect the nucleus solitarius and the nucleus ambiguus. Afferent neural signals from the heart reach the nucleus solitarius with information about the chemical and mechanical conditions in the heart and other organs.

Depending on the nature of that information, a signal is passed on to the nucleus ambiguus to either stimulate the efferent sympathetic nerves to increase heart rate or stimulate the efferent vagal nerve fibers to reduce heart rate. The process of respiration is intimately linked to regulation of the heart's pacemaker by the ANS, with exhalation causing an increased vagal response, known as the "vagal brake" because it slows down the heart. During inhalation, the vagal brake is released, and the heart rate increases because of an underlying sympathetic influence and the natural frequency of the sinoatrial node. Respiratory sinus arrhythmia is the result of this on-off vagal activity.

Respiratory sinus arrhythmia: the detailed mechanisms

We will first consider how the mechanical properties of the cardiovascular (CV) system affect how it reacts during each breath cycle. A diagram of the CV system is shown in Figure 5.3. The systemic veins carry blood back to the heart after the blood has delivered oxygen and nutrients to the organs. At this point, the blood is at a low pressure and so the thin-walled veins are adequate containers. The veins have the capability to dilate, and they act as a reservoir of blood that can be tapped into if the need arises. During inspiration, the chest expands and the pressure within the thorax decreases. This effectively increases the blood pressure within the systemic veins because there is not so much pressure exerted on their outer surface. As a result, more blood flows back to the heart, and "venous return" is increased. The extra blood enters the heart through the right atrium which stretches the wall and activates stretch receptors.

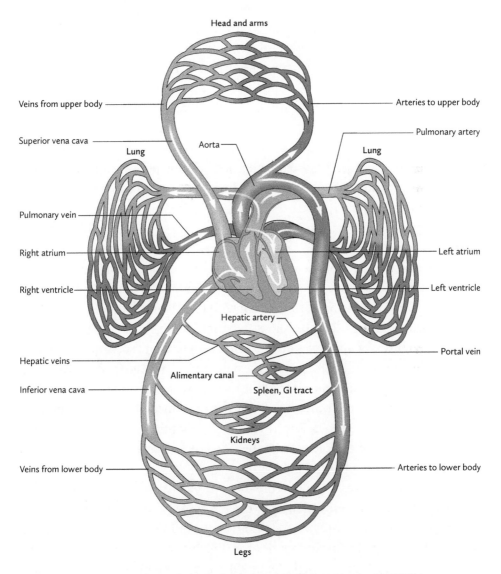

FIGURE 5.3 DIAGRAM OF THE CARDIOVASCULAR SYSTEM.

These receptors send impulses along the afferent vagal fibers to the medulla oblongata in the brain stem, which leads to stimulation of the vasomotor center. As a result, impulses are sent along efferent, sympathetic nerves to the heart and heart rate increases. The increase in heart rate produced by a rise in atrial pressure is known as the "Bainbridge reflex," and it arises because the heart needs to beat faster to transport the extra blood from the pulmonary artery to the lungs where the blood receives oxygen.

On exhalation, oxygenated extra blood from lung circulation enters the left heart and is pumped into the aorta, so arterial pressure temporarily increases. Arterial baroreceptors in the walls of the aortic arch and carotid sinus respond to the increased arterial pressure by instructing the vasomotor center to stimulate efferent vagal nerves to decrease heart rate. That is why heart rate decreases during a long exhale. Another reason for the reduction in heart rate is that intrathoracic pressure increases on the exhale, leading to decreased venous return and less stretching of sensors in the wall of the right atrium. If it were not for these sensitive biofeedback mechanisms, we would not be able to coordinate respiration with HRV and the respiratory component to HRV would remain low.

Benefits of increased RSA

It is reported that pronounced RSA is beneficial to circulation (Bernardi *et al.* 1998, 2001; Friedman and Coats 2000) and improves well-being (Friedman and Coats 2001). Coordination of respiration with HRV benefits the circulation and general health because it increases oxygenation of the blood. As can be seen by studying Figures 5.1 and 5.3, with each inhale, heart rate increases, and extra blood is simultaneously pumped into the pulmonary circulation where it receives oxygen. The extra blood reaches the lungs at the exact same time as there is extra air in the lungs. On the other hand, uneven or reduced RSA is a predictor of circulatory complications (La Rovere *et al.* 1998). For this reason, yogic breathing, which produces pronounced RSA, has beneficial effects on blood pressure (Misra *et al.* 2018) and HRV (Tay and Baldwin 2015).

In the study addressing blood pressure, 83 participants with hypertension (high blood pressure) were divided into three groups. Two of the groups practiced breathing exercises in 15-minute sessions five times a week. One of these groups attended classes led by Misra, and the other followed a DVD/online instructional video. The third group did not participate in the breathing exercises. Participants in the yogic breathing study performed five exercises:

1. Bellow breathing: take deep breaths that fill lungs to the collar bones, followed by deep exhales.
2. Rapid exhalations: in quick bursts, expel air through the nose 10–15 times after each inhalation.

3. Alternate nostril breathing: close right nostril and breathe in through left, then close left nostril and breathe out through right.
4. Bumblebee breathing: plug ears and breathe in and out through nose while humming like a bee.
5. Om singing: breathe in normally and say "Om" while exhaling.

Overall, the people who did the yogic breathing exercises, whether in class or online, were significantly more likely to reduce their systolic blood pressure by at least 5 mmHg compared to people in the control group.

In the study addressing effects of yogic breathing on HRV, 13 students were enrolled into a ten-week vinyasa yoga program and asked to attend at least three of the yoga classes. Vinyasa yoga entails a flow of different poses that are paired with breathing practice. Before and after each class, the students' HRV and respiration rates were measured. For measurements taken before the class, students were asked to breathe the way they usually do when at rest. For post measure-

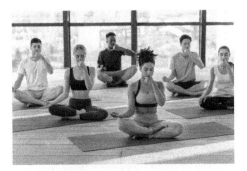

FIGURE 5.4 A YOGA CLASS
PERFORMING ALTERNATE
NOSTRIL BREATHING.
Source: Eva Norlyk Smith.
www.yogauonline.com.

ments, the students continued with the breathing practice used during the yoga class. Heart rate variability was significantly higher after each class than before, but heart rate did not change. Average respiration rate after the last session each student attended was significantly lower than before the session. These results are consistent with relaxation and an increased ability to handle stress.

HOW TO SYNCHRONIZE BREATHING AND HRV TO ACTIVATE THE VAGUS NERVE

Breathing a little more deeply and slowly than usual is probably the easiest and most effective way of activating the vagus nerve. Just exhale! Reap the benefits as envisioned in the following poem by Buddhist monk Thich Nhat Hanh.

Our True Heritage
The cosmos is filled with precious gems.

I want to offer a handful of them to you this morning.
Each moment you are alive is a gem,
shining through and containing earth and sky,
water and clouds.
It needs you to breathe gently
for the miracles to be displayed.
Suddenly you hear the birds singing,
the pines chanting,
see the flowers blooming,
the blue sky,
the white clouds,
the smile and the marvelous look
of your beloved.
You, the richest person on Earth,
who have been going around begging for a living,
stop being the destitute child.
Come back and claim your heritage.
We should enjoy our happiness
and offer it to everyone.
Cherish this very moment.
Let go of the stream of distress
and embrace life fully in your arms.

Source: Call Me By My True Names, The Collected Poems of Thich Nhat Hanh.

There are two breathing practices I use for myself and my clients that I have found to be both enjoyable and effective: Heart-Focused Breathing™ (HFB), developed by the Institute of HeartMath, and Gassho breathing used in Reiki.

Heart-Focused Breathing™

Heart-Focused Breathing™ (HFB) was the initial technique I used with my client who featured in the case study included in Chapter 4, "Shifting to calm with heartfelt gratitude." This type of breathing shifts a person into a state of ANS balance in which sympathetic and parasympathetic nerves interact, or "talk to each other," on a second-by-second basis to enable all physiological systems to function optimally. Problems arise if the sympathetic ANS component takes over on a chronic basis. For example, chronic sympathetic overstimulation puts you continually in the "fight or flight" mode, so you over-react to each small disturbance as if it were a major issue. Your heart rate increases and HRV decreases, leading to reduced vagal activity and increased risk of heart disease (Goldenberg *et al.* 2019). Low HRV is also associated with poor emotional regulation and cognitive function (Cattaneo *et al.* 2021). Instructions for the HFB exercise are shown in Box 5.1.

BOX 5.1 HEART-FOCUSED BREATHING™

During HFB, you focus your attention on your heart or chest area, and, as you breathe, you imagine the breath entering and leaving your heart, while breathing slightly more deeply and slowly than usual.

It might be useful at first to count to five as you inhale, and to five as you exhale, "one and two and three and four and five." If this makes you feel lightheaded or dizzy, reduce the count to three or four.

There is no need to lift your shoulders as you breathe in. This is not a chore. It should feel pleasantly relaxing.

It is usual to breathe in and out through your nose but do whatever is comfortable.

I also find it helps to consciously relax your muscles on every exhale, starting with your toes on your first exhale and ending with your forehead on your last exhale. Do not forget to include your tongue and jaw.

If you find your mind wandering, just focus back on your breathing.

A five-minute practice twice a day works wonders. You will start to feel less drained and more energized and calm at the same time. This is also a useful exercise to do when you feel overwhelmed by a situation and need to take a step back. Often HFB helps you think more clearly and quickly access solutions to the problem at hand. The first time I practiced HFB at the Institute of Heart-Math, Boulder Creek, California, I was walking in the woodlands surrounding the buildings and saw a small deer. I stopped walking and focused on breathing from my heart to the deer's heart, back and forth. The deer made eye contact, walked towards me and stood still, without a trace of fear (Figure 5.5).

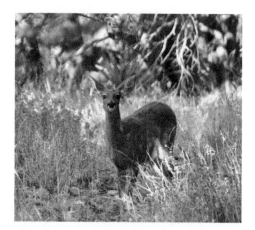

FIGURE 5.5 REACTION OF DEER TO HEART-FOCUSED BREATHING.

Gassho breathing

Gassho breathing was developed by Reiki founder, Mikao Usui and used with his students to bring unity to the body. "Gassho" means "palms placed together in front of the chest" or "prayer position" as shown by the statue in Figure 5.6

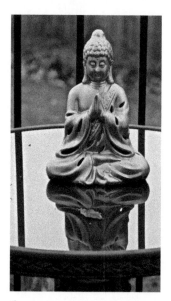

FIGURE 5.6 STATUE OF BUDDHA IN GASSHO.

Gassho breathing is very simple. Similar to HFB, Gassho breathing will keep you calm and energized at the same time. After a few minutes, you will feel clear-headed and ready to face any challenges that may arise. The instructions for Gassho breathing are given in Box 5.2.

BOX 5.2 GASSHO BREATHING

Sit either on the floor or upright in a chair in a relaxed position with your hands in prayer position.

Concentrate on breathing in and out slowly through your nose (about five seconds in and five seconds out).

With each in-breath, imagine that Reiki energy is entering your crown and filling your entire body. For those of you who are not trained in Reiki, imagine light entering your crown and filling your entire body.

With each out-breath, visualize that you are exhaling Reiki (or light) from every pore in your body and off out to infinity.

SOME PERSONAL EXPERIENCES

Ann L. Baldwin, PhD, Physiologist, HeartMath Certified Trainer, Usui Reiki Master, Mind-Body-Science (abaldwin@mind-body-science.com)

The power of breathing to gain inner clarity

One way to quickly stimulate your vagus nerve is to take a few deep breaths. As you exhale, your vagus nerve releases acetylcholine which slows down the heart and puts the body into "rest and digest" mode. Since most of us are usually over-aroused as we try to fit as much as we can into the day, we often forget this simple truth. It gets even worse if you are having to cope with unexpected roadblocks that are flung in your way. But it is worth remembering that cultivating the release of those squirts of acetylcholine as needed will bring you into coherence and give you clarity. I found that skill very useful when a friend looked at a gift that I had given them.

I realized from their expression, similar to that shown in Figure 5.7, that it was not right for them. Instead of getting over-aroused and upset, I focused on my heart, took a few deep breaths, relaxed my face and was immediately able to think clearly. I remembered that I'd saved the receipt, where I had put it, and I looked forward to going with my friend to return the gift and exchange it for something they really wanted. Of course, it does take practice to remember to stop, sense your heart and adjust your breathing right there in the present moment, but it is worth it!

The power of breathing to banish frustration

I was returning from a conference, "Horses and Humans," in North Carolina. It was wonderful to hear about the stories and supporting data from other researchers and equine professionals about all the

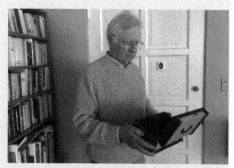

FIGURE 5.7 EXPRESSION OF DISAPPOINTMENT.

ways that horses can help us self-regulate. For example, magnetic resonance imaging brain scans taken of military veterans before and after they participated in an equine-assisted learning program over several weeks showed that the part of the brain responsible for their reward reaction became better connected to other parts of the brain, meaning that they could experience joy and pleasure at a more conscious level.

My journey home taught me something else: the importance of being able to effectively self-regulate when I was in danger of getting so mad that my body would be damaged by the release of inappropriate hormones and neurotransmitters. That was because after entering the airport I encountered a totally confused mob and I was unable to find out what to do. Instead of joining the fray, I stood still, focused on my heart and imagined the breath going into my heart on the inhale and out of my heart on the exhale. With every exhale, I consciously relaxed all my muscles from my toes to my forehead, including my eyes and my tongue.

After a few moments, I looked around and discovered that I needed to join a slowly moving, snaking line to get through the Transportation Security Administration pre-check. It took 90 minutes, and that was in the fast lane. I do not like queues and avoid them whenever possible, but this time I had no choice. Most people were desperately tapping on their cell phones, for what reason I have no idea, because it did not get them through any more quickly. I kept things simple and just focused on my heart breath and relaxing my muscles. We eventually boarded the plane and were ready to go. Success! But no. We had to wait another two hours on the runway because the caterers had not yet loaded the special food on the plane for the first-class passengers. By that time, I decided I needed a change, so I focused on imagining inhaling through my crown until the breath reached just above my navel, and then exhaling through every pore of my body. I am glad to say that worked and I avoided getting anxious, frustrated and sick.

LAUGHTER YOGA

When did you last laugh heartily? The Association for Applied and Therapeutic Humor indicates that, on average, adults laugh about 20 times a day, but the number can range from zero to 80. According to the Mayo Clinic, laughter has many short- and long-term health benefits, listed below.

Short-term effects:

- Stimulates many organs. Laughter enhances your intake of oxygen-rich air, stimulates your heart, lungs and muscles, and increases the endorphins that are released by your brain.
- Activates and relieves your stress response. A rollicking laugh fires up and then cools down your stress response, and it can increase and then decrease your heart rate and blood pressure. The result? A good, relaxed feeling.
- Soothes tension. Laughter can also stimulate circulation and aid muscle relaxation, both of which can help reduce some of the physical symptoms of stress.

Long-term effects:

- Improves your immune system. Negative thoughts manifest into chemical reactions that can affect your body by bringing more stress into your system and decreasing your immunity. By contrast, positive thoughts can actually release neuropeptides that help fight stress and potentially more serious illnesses.

- Relieves pain. Laughter may ease pain by causing the body to produce its own natural painkillers.
- Increases personal satisfaction. Laughter can also make it easier to cope with difficult situations. It also helps you connect with other people.
- Improves your mood. Many people experience depression, sometimes due to chronic illnesses. Laughter can help lessen your stress, depression and anxiety, and may make you feel happier. It can also improve your self-esteem.

Activation of pulmonary, cardiac, laryngeal and facial vagus nerve branches

The short- and long-term benefits of laughter can be traced back in large part to stimulation of the vagus nerve. The pulmonary branch of the vagus nerve is activated with every burst of exhales that accompanies laughter, the laryngeal branches are activated by making the sounds of laughter, and the facial branches by engaging the facial muscles that control the corner of the mouth with a lateral upward movement, or smile. The cardiovascular vagal branches, on the other hand, are not very activated by laughter, at least at the beginning. Instead, the sympathetic cardiac nerves are stimulated, leading to a temporary increase in heart rate and a reduction in HRV, rather like physical exercise (Law *et al.* 2018). This response leads to improved blood circulation which benefits the heart and the muscles.

Mirthful laughter, which is that caused by merriment and jollity, induces the release of β-endorphins, leading to release of nitric oxide. Nitric oxide relaxes the walls of small blood vessels called arterioles, causing them to dilate, deliver more blood to the tissues and reduce blood pressure. Nitric oxide may also reduce vascular inflammation (Miller and Fry 2009). Because laughing involves such a complicated array of muscles and physiological systems, vigorous laughing is thought to relax muscles, improve respiration and circulation, and decrease the production of stress-related hormones in the brain (Martin 2002).

A popular way to combine laughter with deep breathing techniques is through laughter yoga. This practice dates back to 1995 when Dr Madan Kataria, a family physician, assembled a small group of people in a public park in Mumbai, who met each morning to laugh together through a series of funny expressions and movements that Dr Kataria developed. Nearly 30 years later, more than 15,000 laughter yoga clubs exist in more than 70 countries worldwide. Figure 5.8 shows a typical scene from a laughter yoga class.

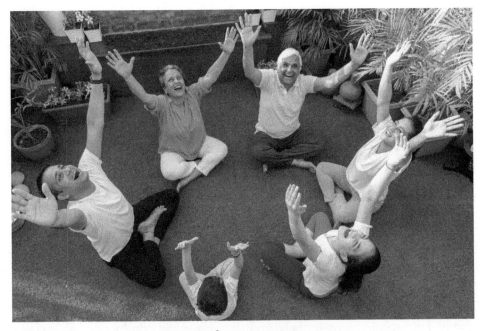

FIGURE 5.8 LAUGHTER YOGA.

A typical laughter yoga session lasts from 30 to 60 minutes, during which a leader engages participants in a series of movements and breathing exercises designed to promote forced laughter that converts to spontaneous laughter as the session wears on. Most sessions begin with simple breathing techniques, clapping and chanting to help people relax. For example, you might begin the class by clapping rhythmically 1-2, 1-2-3 while chanting "ho-ho, ha-ha-ha." The session may also include gentle stretching, yoga breath work and meditation.

Research in the field of laughter yoga is currently sparse and includes only small studies. For example, Dolgoff-Kaspar *et al.* (2012) evaluated the clinical utility of laughter yoga in improving psychological and physiological outcomes in six patients awaiting organ (heart or lung) transplantation. The study started with a control period of one week during which the participants spent 20 minutes discussing health and study-related topics with the investigators at the beginning and end of the week. After the control period, participants completed seven 20-minute laughter yoga sessions over a period of three weeks. These sessions involved breathing and stretching exercises, simulated laughter, chanting, clapping and a meditation. Participants showed improved immediate mood (vigor-activity and friendliness) and increased HRV after the laughter yoga. Both the laughter and control interventions appeared to improve longer-term anxiety. Considering the small sample size and limited follow-up period, the results

Considering the small sample size and limited follow-up period, the results should be interpreted with caution. Nevertheless, the findings are encouraging and suggest the need for further research.

A 2019 review (van der Wal and Kok 2019) found simulated laughter lowered depression rates and improved mood. In fact, simulated laughter was more effective than spontaneous laughter. Other studies have shown that laughter yoga may help temporarily reduce concentration of the stress hormone, cortisol, improve mood and energy levels, and induce a more positive mindset (Miles *et al.* 2016; Yazdani *et al.* 2014). Laughter yoga may even be as effective as aerobic exercise at reducing self-reported stress (Shahidi *et al.* 2010). These encouraging results from small-scale studies support the development of clinical trials in which laughter therapy is one component of an integrated therapeutic lifestyle program.

One factor missing from most of the discussion about the health-promoting effectiveness of laughter yoga is the aspect of laughing with other people. Laughing in a group can increase social connectedness and bonding and strengthen relationships. It is also linked to feelings of security and safety, allowing a person to feel more relaxed (Kurtz and Algoe 2015; Manninen *et al.* 2017). A quote from Rumi makes the point that you can use the power of your heart to bring out the best in others:

> I have come to drag you out of yourself and take you into my heart. I have come to bring out the beauty you never knew you had and lift you like a prayer to the sky.

Perhaps that is what is happening when people get together in a group and just laugh.

To conclude, a short meditation focusing on breathing a little more slowly and deeply than usual is one of the easiest and most effective ways to stimulate the vagus nerve. Vagal stimulation by breath regulation works through the pulmonary branches. There is abundant scientific evidence that this activity enhances physical, mental and emotional health. Laughter yoga, on the other hand, is a much more complex therapy than breath regulation for several reasons. First, it involves multiple routes for accessing the vagus nerve including the pulmonary, laryngeal and facial branches. Second, it is not purely a relaxation technique because it also stimulates the cardiac sympathetic nerves, increasing heart rate and blood circulation, similar to exercise. Third, it is usually practiced in a group setting and so evokes social engagement which often brings other benefits. Some exercises are performed in pairs which requires that the participants develop feelings of trust and collaboration. This can only be achieved in the presence of adequate vagal stimulation. For these reasons, it may take multiple sessions before participants feel comfortable in a class and can reap the benefits. Although there is presently a sparsity of scientific evidence in support of laughter yoga, the existing results are promising, and larger studies are clearly warranted.

CASE STUDY: Laughing through pain and anxiety
Laura Key, LMT, MS, Founder of Lotus Massage & Wellness Center, Tucson, AZ

The intentional and regular practice of laughter offers an intriguing demonstration of the profound benefits that can result from stimulation of the vagus nerve even in the face of serious physical and emotional challenges. The case of MM is the story of an individual using laughter to treat complex regional pain syndrome (CRPS), considered by physicians to be the most painful condition known to humankind.

CRPS is a chronic disease of unknown cause and with no known cure. This rare pain dysfunction syndrome causes inflammation and pain often described by patients as constant, burning, intense, severe, unbearable. Although there is no definitive cause, researchers believe the sympathetic nervous system may be involved in some way. There may have been a previous injury, but if so, the area with pain is more extensive than that injury, such as an entire limb.

In any case, CRPS pain persists long beyond a normal recovery period and the level of pain is wholly out of proportion to any earlier injury. Light touch or even moving air can trigger extreme pain. Whole-body symptoms can include abnormal sweating. Complex regional pain syndrome usually causes significant emotional distress characterized by difficulty concentrating, insomnia, depression and anxiety.

MM had explored laughter yoga before ending up as a CRPS patient, but CRPS influenced her to make laughter a regular part of her daily life. Her doctors had prescribed narcotic painkillers, and she was weak and ill but trying to taper off her usage. She decided to start trying to laugh throughout her day, for a full hour total, using both conventional laughter and laughter yoga.

Conventional laughter is relatively passive in origin and is sourced externally. It reflects cultural expectations and norms and relies on humor occurring in jokes, wit, comedy or circumstances. Specifically, conventional laughter relies on mental cognizance of humorous cues to trigger the physical act of laughter. Laughter yoga involves laughter without the usual external triggers. Dr. Madan

Kataria, MD, the Mumbai-based founder of the international laughter yoga movement, calls it "the art of laughing for no reason." It requires an intentional and creative act, with the laughter sourced internally via conscious decision.

Laughter yoga is "yoga" in the sense that it uses focused attention and integrates stretching, other body movement, chanting and the same breathing principles as traditional yoga. Good eye contact with others is encouraged in laughter yoga clubs or groups. At each session, participants engage in a series of varying "laughter exercises" intended to reduce inhibitions and generate a sense of childlike playfulness, even childlike joy. Hundreds of these exercises have been devised. Examples include belly-holding ho-ho-ho laughter, knee-slapping heehaw laughter, maniacal wicked witch laughter, finger-to-lips silent laughter, roaring lion laughter, handshake meet-and-greet laughter, pointing to and laughing at one's physical pains, or play-acting that one is on a cell call with someone who is hysterically funny while gesturing at the imaginary phone and shrugging.

During each exercise, participants make a choice to engage in the facial expressions, physical movements and sounds of laughter. The movements or acting out of each exercise combine with eye contact and the sounds of others to help some participants shift toward unconditional laughter. However, it is not considered a concern that other participants continue using simulated laughter.

Some might construe externally sourced passive laughter as "real" and internally sourced simulated laughter as "fake," but the difference is immaterial. The body does not distinguish. Natural and simulated laughter both involve a characteristic facial expression with the ends of the mouth turned up, comparable use of the vocal cords, comparable activity of the lungs, and otherwise similar physical actions. Research has shown the physiological outcomes and health benefits of both types of laughter to be the same.

While to many people laughter is a group activity, MM often employs laughter alone at home. Originally, she relied on laughter yoga videos posted online. She also tried laughter yoga groups but felt shy in that setting. With practice, MM internalized laughter yoga principles and grew her ability to transition easily from simulated laughter to natural laughter. She also watches stand-up comedy and other comedy shows, and uses jokes, at times simply telling jokes to herself, sometimes entertaining companions. Thus, she uses a combination of active and passive laughter.

Besides laughing solo, MM laughs with her boyfriend. She allows that "Chronic pain can make you kind of touchy" and admits that at times she has started "a ridiculous argument over nothing" with him. But they are both able to use laughter to defuse such situations, with one or the other breaking into a loud silly laugh, which reminds and triggers the other to laugh, and they then laugh together until the argument is behind them.

Her CRPS has caused extreme night sweats, with MM waking drenched, sometimes in a full-blown anxiety attack. She describes crying and sobbing in despair but then remembering a laughter yoga exercise that includes mock sobbing as well as mock laughter. She presses herself to laugh in as many ways as she can think of until her pounding pulse drops and she feels grounded and safe.

MM uses the classic phrase "the best medicine" to describe laughter. Beyond its benefits in her own life, she has witnessed its benefits in the life of her partner, a US Marine who suffers from post-traumatic stress disorder (PTSD), and in the life of her father, who died of health conditions caused by Agent Orange exposure but lived a year longer than doctors expected – a year filled with laughter.

MM credits laughter as helping her move beyond both her pain and anxiety.

I could not survive this without the ability to laugh even at the most horrific moments... After laughing I feel like I can survive, like I can make it through the day and have fun even though...remission is impossible. Laughter helps to bring us present, in this moment, right now, which is not only helpful for chronic pain but for life in general.

REFERENCES

Bernardi L, Spadacini G, Bellwon J et al., 1998. Effect of breathing rate on oxygen saturation and exercise performance in chronic heart failure. *Lancet.* 351: 1308–1311. doi: 10.1016/S0140-6736(97)10341.

Bernardi L, Sleight P, Bandinelli G et al., 2001. Effect of rosary prayer and yoga mantras on autonomic cardiovascular rhythms: comparative study. *British Medical Journal.* 323(7327): 1446–1449. doi: 10.1136/bmj.323.7327.1446.

Cattaneo LA, Franquillo AC, Grecucci A et al., 2021. Is low heart rate variability associated with emotional dysregulation, psychopathological dimensions, and prefrontal dysfunctions? An integrative view. *J Pers Med.* 11(9): 872. doi: 10.3390/jpm11090872.

Dolgoff-Kaspar R, Baldwin A, Johnson MS et al., 2012. Effect of laughter yoga on mood and heart rate variability in patients awaiting organ transplantation: a pilot study. *Alternative Therapies.* 18: 4.

Friedman EH and Coats AJ, 2000. Neurobiology of exaggerated heart oscillations during two meditative techniques. *Int J Cardiol.* 73: 199. doi: 10.1016/S0167-5273(00)00214-X.

Goldenberg I, Goldkorn R, Shlomo N et al., 2019. Heart rate variability for risk assessment of myocardial ischemia in patients without known coronary artery disease: the HRV-DETECT (Heart Rate Variability for the Detection of Myocardial Ischemia) study. *Journal of the American Heart Association*. 8: 24. doi: 10.1161/JAHA.119.014540.

Kurtz LE and Algoe SB, 2015. Putting laughter in context: shared laughter as behavioral indicator of relationship well-being. *Pers Relatsh*. 22(4): 573–590. doi: 10.1111/pere.12095.

La Rovere MT, Bigger JT Jr, Marcus FI et al., 1998. Baroreflex sensitivity and heart-rate variability in prediction of total cardiac mortality after myocardial infarction. ATRAMI (Autonomic Tone and Reflexes After Myocardial Infarction) Investigators. *Lancet*. 351: 478–484. doi: 0.1016/S0140-6736(97)11144-8.

Law MM, Broadbent EA and Sollers JJ, 2018. A comparison of the cardiovascular effects of simulated and spontaneous laughter. *Complementary Therapies in Medicine*. 37: 103–109. doi: 10.1016/j.ctim.2018.02.005.

Lehrer PM and Gevirtz R, 2014. Heart rate variability biofeedback. How and why does it work? *Frontiers in Psychology*. 5: 756. doi: 10.3389/fpsyg.2014.00756.

Manninen S, Tuominen L, Dunbar RI et al., 2017. Social laughter triggers endogenous opioid release in humans. *J Neurosci*. 37(25): 6125–6131. doi: 10.1523/JNEUROSCI.0688-16.2017.

Martin RA, 2002. Is laughter the best medicine? Humor, laughter, and physical health. *Current Directions in Psychological Science*. 11(6): 216–220.

Miles C, Tait E, Schure MB and Hollis M, 2016. Effect of laughter yoga on psychological well-being and physiological measures. *Adv Mind Body Med*. 30(1):12–20.

Miller M and Fry WF, 2009. The effect of mirthful laughter on the human cardiovascular system. *Medical Hypotheses*. 73(5): 636–639.

Misra S, Smith J, Wareg N et al., 2018. Take a deep breath: a randomized control trial of Pranayama breathing on uncontrolled hypertension. *Advances in Integrative Medicine*. 6(2): 2018. doi: 10.1016/j.aimed.2018.08.002.

Shahidi M, Mojtahed A, Modabbernia A et al., 2010. Laughter yoga versus group exercise program in elderly depressed women: a randomized controlled trial. *Int J Geriatr Psychiatry*. 3: 322–327. doi: 10.1002/gps.2545.

Song HS and Lehrer PM, 2003. The effects of specific respiratory rates on heart rate and heart rate variability. *Appl Psychophysiol Biofeedback*. 28: 13–23. doi: 10.1023/A:1022312815649.

Sukhova GS and Mazurov ME, 2007. Mechanical-electrical processes involved in the synchronization of the sinus node from atria. *Doklady Biochemistry and Biophysics*. 412(1): 22–24. doi: 10.1134/S1607672907010073.

Tay K and Baldwin AL, 2015. Effects of breathing practice in Vinyasa yoga on heart rate variability in university students – a pilot study. *Journal of Yoga & Physical Therapy*. 5: 4. doi: 10.4172/2157-7595.1000214.

van der Wal CN and Kok RN, 2019. Laughter-inducing therapies: systematic review and meta-analysis. *Soc Sci Med*. 232: 473–488. doi: 10.1016/j.socscimed.2019.02.018.

Yazdani M, Esmaeilzadeh M, Pahlavanzadeh S and Khaledi F, 2014. The effect of laughter yoga on general health among nursing students. *Iran J Nurs Midwifery Res*. 1: 36–40.

CHAPTER 6

Abdominal and Intestinal Branches

DIGESTION, DIET AND THE MICROBIOME

INTRODUCTION

The common name for the vagal, or parasympathetic, component of the auto-nomic nervous system (ANS) is "rest and digest." This is the state when cell repair and healing take place. Many people spend most of their waking moments dwelling on the past or worrying about the future. These states activate your sympathetic nervous system and take you out of the "rest and digest" mode. This sympathetic dominance causes a weakening of the parasympathetic rest-digest-heal response, so many people are unable to activate it effectively when they need it. One of the major functions of the vagus system is to control diges-tion. As seen in Figure 6.1, the gastric branches of the vagus nerve innervate the stomach, and the intestinal and abdominal branches innervate the small and large intestine. These nerves convey messages between the gut and the brain.

In this chapter we will learn about the details of gut-brain and brain-gut communication, focusing on the enteric nervous system which is the part of the ANS devoted to the intestine. We will also discuss the importance of the microbiome, the bacteria lining the inner surface of the intestine, and how they influence communication between the gut and the brain in both directions. Due to the dense neural connection between the intestine and the brain, you will see that digestion affects mood, and mood affects digestion. Even the little bacteria in your gut can influence your mood.

Most of this chapter will focus on how you can improve your digestion and your mood by participating in activities that stimulate vagal activity in the gut. These include:

- Eating high-quality food with friends: rest, digest and engage.
- Colon hydrotherapy with massage and breathwork to stimulate your vagus nerve and improve digestion.
- Treating damaged vagus nerve and impaired gastric emptying (gastro-paresis) with acupuncture.
- Culturing your gut microbiota to reduce anxiety and improve mood.

These activities will improve gut function by optimizing the intestinal chemical environment and the mechanical stresses to which the gut is exposed, and will also improve your mood and lessen psychiatric disorders and depression as visualized in Figure 6.1.

AUTONOMIC NERVOUS CONNECTION BETWEEN BRAIN AND INTESTINE

The vagal efferent fibers (10–20% of all fibers) send signals from the brain to the gut, and the afferent fibers (80–90% of all fibers), from the walls of the stomach and intestine to the brain. Efferent fibers regulate the contraction of smooth muscles in the muscular (myenteric) layers of the gut to stimulate propulsion of food along the length of the intestine and regulate glandular secretion of gastric acid and digestive enzymes in the inner, mucosal layers of the gut. Preganglionic neurons of vagal efferent fibers emerge from the dorsal motor nucleus in the medulla.

Afferent fibers in the walls of the stomach and intestine receive information about the chemical environment in the gut from chemoreceptors that reside mainly in the mucosa. Information about tension in the walls of the stomach and intestine comes from mechanoreceptors and tension receptors located mainly in the muscular layers. If you have just eaten a large meal, you will feel full because your stomach walls stretch, and the tension receptors will be stimulated. If you are hungry, this will elicit the opposite effect. If you eat too much of a food that might cause inflammation, such as processed meat, the immune cells in the gut inner lining will be activated to release substances such as cytokines that may cause tissue damage, and this response will be detected by chemoreceptors. All this information is sent up to the sensory afferent cell bodies in the nodose ganglia to the nucleus tractus solitarius (NTS). The NTS projects the vagal sensory information to several regions of the brain, such as the locus coeruleus (LC), the amygdala and the thalamus. That is how your brain knows what is going on in your gut.

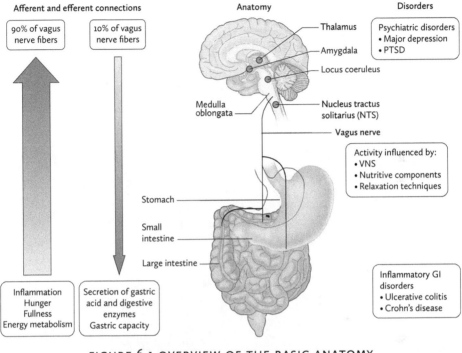

FIGURE 6.1 OVERVIEW OF THE BASIC ANATOMY
AND FUNCTIONS OF THE VAGUS NERVE.
NTS, nucleus tractus solitarius; VNS, vagus nerve stimulation.
Source: Adapted from Breit et al. 2018, Figure 1.

One important system not shown in Figure 6.1 is the microbiome, defined as the community of microorganisms, such as bacteria, viruses and fungi, in the environment. When considering the microorganisms living in one specific location such as the inner mucosal surface of the gut, the term used is microbiota. When you digest food, the vagus nerve endings in the gut sense changes in the microbiota in your intestines and send this information to your brain (Figure 6.2).

When the vagus nerve is working correctly, the brain sends back the right response immediately. For example, if you eat a food that triggers intestinal inflammation, the mucosal chemoreceptors detect cytokines that are released by the neighboring activated immune cells. The receptors send this information to the brain via the vagal afferent fibers in the mucosal nerves: "Hey, brain. There's some inflammation here. Do something!" The brain then sends information back to the intestine, initiating a biological process that decreases the inflammation.

For example, the efferent mucosal vagus nerve endings might be stimulated to produce the neurotransmitter, acetylcholine, which then binds to the immune cells to inhibit them from releasing the cytokines that produce inflammation.

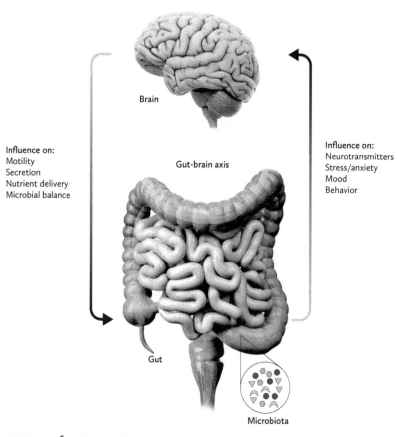

Brain

Influence on:
Motility
Secretion
Nutrient delivery
Microbial balance

Gut-brain axis

Influence on:
Neurotransmitters
Stress/anxiety
Mood
Behavior

Gut

Microbiota

FIGURE 6.2 THE GUT-BRAIN-MICROBIOME CONNECTION.

The microbiota in the gut can also affect our mood and emotions. For example, gut bacteria manufacture about 95 percent of the body's supply of serotonin, which not only increases the activity of the gastrointestinal system but also influences psychological mood. Species of *Bifidobacterium*, *Lactobacillus* (lactic acid bacteria) and *Lactococcus* often exist in the colon where they exert a positive influence on anxiety and stress. The microbiota alone is not responsible for these effects on mood. They only occur in the presence of a well-functioning vagus nerve. The influence of the microbiota on mood is not a one-way street. Your mood can also alter the microbiota. Even mild stress can change the microbial balance in the gut, making you more vulnerable to infectious disease. These important topics will be addressed in more detail later in the chapter.

REST, DIGEST AND ENGAGE

The intestine's own nervous system (enteric system)

The gut has its own nervous system, the enteric nervous system (ENS), which contains about 500 million neurons (about the same number as in the spinal cord), produces 40 known neurotransmitters (the brain produces 100) and produces 50 percent of the body's dopamine and 95 percent of the serotonin. For this reason, the gut is often termed "the second brain," although it is not capable of conscious thought or decision making. The brain and ENS can be compared to a computer network, with the brain being a main frame computer, and the ENS a laptop or iPad.

The ENS consists of sheaths of neurons embedded in the walls of the alimentary canal, which measures about nine meters (the width of three lanes of highway) end to end from the esophagus to the anus. It takes care of the processes of digestion (breaking down food, absorbing nutrients and expelling of waste) on its own, without the need for the brain or spinal cord. Therefore, the ENS can integrate information received from the sensory neurons and act on it, unlike other sensory systems. The way in which the ENS relates to the central nervous system (brain and spinal cord) and to the ANS is shown in Figure 6.3.

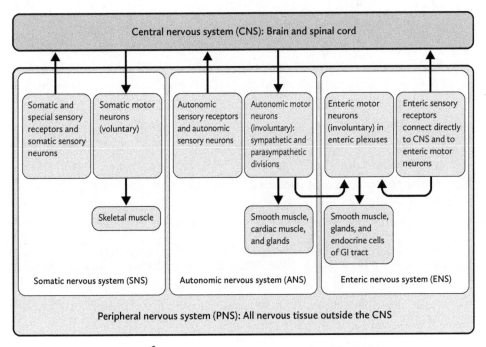

FIGURE 6.3 CONNECTIONS BETWEEN CENTRAL, AUTONOMIC AND ENTERIC NERVOUS SYSTEMS.
Source: © John Wiley and Sons, Inc.

Three subsystems feed into the CNS: the somatic, which serves skeletal muscles; the autonomic, which serves the internal organs; and the ENS, which is really part of the ANS but is shown separately because, unlike the somatic system and the rest of the ANS, the motor and sensory neurons of the ENS are directly connected. That means that information can be sensed and acted upon *without any input from the brain.* Sensory neurons serving other organs do *not* connect directly to the motor neurons and so in these cases the brain needs to be involved in every process. The brain is informed of processes taking place in the gut through the enteric sensory neurons, and it can intervene, if necessary, through the sympathetic and parasympathetic nerves that feed into the motor neurons of the ENS. The gastrointestinal tract also receives a good supply of afferent (sensory) nerve fibers through the vagus nerves and spinal afferent pathways, so there is a rich interaction between the ENS and CNS.

How the vagus nerve controls digestion: gut motility and intestinal secretions

The ENS consists of two nerve plexuses that contain nerve cell bodies, the myenteric plexus that controls peristalsis and churning of intestinal contents by means of motor neurons that activate intestinal muscles, and the submucosal plexus that controls secretion and absorption of digestive enzymes, and local blood flow. The anatomy of these plexuses is shown in Figure 6.4.

The brain sends signals to the gut via sympathetic and parasympathetic (vagal) systems via a small number of "command neurons," which synapse onto the ENS plexuses. Command neurons control the pattern of activity in the gut. The vagus nerve generally stimulates peristalsis and secretion of the gut by release of the neurotransmitters serotonin and acetylcholine. Acetylcholine also relaxes sphincter muscles. The sympathetic nerves (celiac, superior and inferior mesenteric) generally inhibit motor and secretory function and reduce blood flow to the gut by release of the neurotransmitter norepinephrine.

When you are in "fight or flight" mode, the sympathetic nerves are activated, and the digestive system is temporarily shut down to conserve energy for coping with the challenge you are facing. You usually do not feel hungry, and this is not the time to eat a large meal. If you suffer from chronic stress and you need to eat, it can be helpful to take a few deep, slow breaths, focusing on the exhale, prior to eating. This will stimulate the vagus nerve and shift you to the "rest and digest" mode to prepare you for your meal.

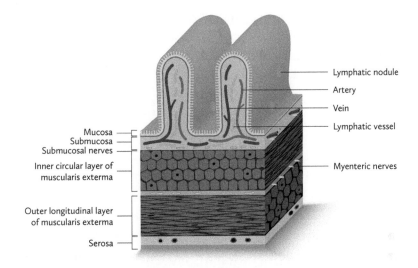

Lymphatic nodule

Artery

Vein

Lymphatic vessel

Myenteric nerves

Mucosa
Submucosa
Submucosal nerves

Inner circular layer of
muscularis exterma

Outer longitudinal layer
of muscularis exterma

Serosa

FIGURE 6.4 THE ENTERIC PLEXUSES OF THE SMALL INTESTINE.
Nerve cells are represented by black circles in the ganglia of the myenteric
and submucosal plexuses. The lines represent nerve fibers innervating
the muscle, villi of the mucosa, arterioles and ganglia.

How a good meal makes you relax

The first sign of a good meal is the aroma. As mentioned in Chapter 2, when we savor an aroma, the olfactory nerve is stimulated. The olfactory nerve is a cranial nerve that forms part of the ventral vagal complex, and so when it is activated, it contributes to the parasympathetic response. But there are several other areas in the brain that are stimulated at the same time, so the overall effect of an aroma on the ANS depends on additional factors and may not necessarily be relaxing.

The smell area of the brain (olfactory cortex), the memory area (hippocampus) and the emotional area (amygdala) are very close to each other. In fact, the olfactory nerve connects directly to the amygdala. This means that a smell can suddenly evoke an emotion or a memory even faster than a sight can because the visual cortex is further away from those areas than is the olfactory cortex. For example, the smell of cabbage reminds me of the unpleasant, overcooked vegetables I had for school dinners and does not shift me to a relaxed "rest and digest" state at all. It is our life experiences that ultimately decide how the aroma affects us emotionally. It seems that scents that make us happier are very specific to the individual. On the other hand, many people share similar scent memories that could be linked to happiness. Many common ingredients can enhance mood and increase feelings of happiness or relaxation.

Regarding food, most people enjoy the aroma of freshly baked bread. This smell not only stimulates the olfactory nerve, but also may evoke nostalgic memories, via the hippocampus, perhaps of friends and family receiving freshly baked bread served straight from the oven. The aroma and memories lead to feelings of security and comfort evoked via the amygdala, resulting in a marked activation of the vagus nerve and a shift to the "rest and digest" state. As you smell the aroma, you will breathe more slowly and deeply to maximize the effect, leading to even greater vagal stimulation with every exhale, as explained in Chapter 5. Vagal stimulation will also activate the salivary glands by means of the glossopharyngeal cranial nerve, to help you lubricate and swallow that first delicious bite. As you chew, the trigeminal and facial cranial nerves will be stimulated, adding further to the vagal shift.

As the food enters the esophagus, the food bolus stretches its walls and activates vagal afferent nerves to signal back to the nucleus tractus solitarius (NTS) that food is present. The multiple neural sympathetic and parasympathetic pathways by which the brain and the gut interact are shown in Figure 6.5. It is evident that there is direct communication to and from the effector systems of the gut (smooth muscle, secretory cells, blood vessels) and the brain stem and limbic system (central autonomic neural network) through both sympathetic and parasympathetic pathways. It is thought that vagal (parasympathetic) afferents are involved in physiological regulation while spinal sympathetic afferents are responsible for mediating pain in diseases such as inflammatory bowel disease. There is also direct communication between the ENS and the effector systems, bypassing the brain.

Currently, it is thought that the signals from sensory fibers in the gastrointestinal tract are received in the NTS and conveyed to the dorsal vagal nucleus to activate vagal motor nerves so that they release acetylcholine and serotonin to promote waves of smooth muscle cell contractions (peristalsis) to push the food downward to the stomach (Herman *et al.* 2009). The celiac branch of the vagus nerve also stimulates release of digestive enzymes from the pancreas and bile from the liver to break down the food so that it can be absorbed. When the food reaches the stomach, hydrochloric acid and pepsin are released to help break down the food even further. Along the way, the celiac nerve regulates the contraction and relaxation of sphincter muscles so that the food continues to move at the right speed and in the right direction as it enters and leaves the stomach.

As the food reaches the small intestine, the abdominal and intestinal branches of the vagus nerve also regulate peristalsis and enzyme secretion. The mechanical force produced by peristalsis stimulates sensors on special cells (enterochromaffin cells) located along the inner surface of the gut wall, to release even more serotonin. It has been shown, at least in rats, that the released serotonin acts on nearby afferent vagal nerve endings to activate vagal nodose neurons to sustain peristalsis and enzyme secretion for digestion (Zhu *et al.* 2001). By now, you are truly in the "rest and digest" state. You consciously recognize that state because the NTS projects the vagal sensory information to the amygdala and the thalamus in the limbic system (Berthoud and Neuhuber 2000) and those structures send the information to the prefrontal cortex, the cognitive, or "thinking," part of the brain.

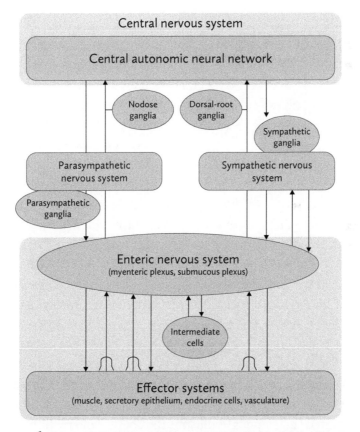

FIGURE 6.5 NEURAL CONNECTIONS BETWEEN BRAIN AND GUT.
Intermediate cells are cells within the mucosal wall, such as
enterochromaffin cells, that stimulate the ENS.
Source: Prins 2011, Figure 2. Used by permission of Taylor & Francis.

If you are eating your meal with good friends, then according to the polyvagal theory, your vagus nerve may become even more stimulated. As described in Chapter 1, the ventral vagus is neuroanatomically linked to the cranial nerves that promote social engagement via eye contact, facial expression and vocalization. This association of the vagus and other cranial nerves, termed the "ventral vagal complex," facilitates hearing, eating, speech, singing, kissing and smiling, which are all part of social engagement. Being relaxed makes it easier to enjoy your friends' company because you are not rushing to do the next thing on your list. So social engagement with good friends will add to your vagal stimulation and shift you even more into the "rest and digest" state (Figure 6.6).

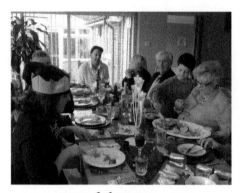

FIGURE 6.6 REST, DIGEST AND ENGAGE.

In case you are worried that you will eat too much and become overweight, your vagus nerve will take care of you if it is functioning appropriately. If you have optimal vagus nerve function and tone, you will easily recognize when you are full because stretch-sensitive vagal neurons in the stomach, and some parts of the intestine, become stimulated and transmit that information to the NTS (Bai *et al.* 2019). Due to the abundance of neural connectivity between the brain stem, the limbic system and the prefrontal cortex, it does not take very long for you to become conscious of the feeling of satiation.

It takes about 20 minutes after you start eating for the message to stop eating to form and reach your brain, says registered dietitian Joanne V. Lichten, author of *Dining Lean: How to Eat Healthy When You're Not at Home*. Nevertheless, it is important to be mindful not only of how much you are eating but also *what* you are eating, and not to rely on the process of digestion as your sole means of stimulating your vagus nerve to relax. Beware of sugar. According to researcher Diego V. Bohórquez: "When we ingest sugar, it stimulates cells in the gut, and these cells release glutamate and activate the vagus nerve" (Buchanan *et al.* 2022). Bohórquez and his team observed that these gut sensor cells, which the team named "neuropods," transmit the chemosensory information to the vagus nerve mere milliseconds after detecting sugar. This response can lead to "emotional eating," in which sweet, fatty foods are craved to reduce feelings of stress. There is evidence to suggest that diets high in added sugar promote the development of metabolic disease, cardiovascular disease and type 2 diabetes (Stanhope 2016).

So, eating is an easy way to stimulate your vagus nerve on a daily basis, but please remember to be judicious in your food choices. According to Jan

Chozen Bays (Zen teacher, author and pediatrician), mindful eating helps you to eat in a balanced way (Bays 2009). If you've heard about mindful eating but aren't sure where or how to start, here are instructions for a brief mindfulness eating exercise (Box 6.1). The following exercise is simple and will only take a few minutes.

BOX 6.1 A MINDFULNESS EATING EXERCISE: SIMPLE INSTRUCTIONS

Find a small piece of food, such as one raisin or nut, or a small cookie. You can use any food that you like. Eating with mindfulness is not about deprivation or rules.

Begin by exploring this little piece of food, using as many of your senses as possible. First, look at the food. Notice its texture. Notice its color.

Now, close your eyes and explore the food with your sense of touch. What does this food feel like? Is it hard or soft? Grainy or sticky? Moist or dry?

Notice that you're not being asked to think but just to notice different aspects of your experience, using one sense at a time. This is what it means to eat mindfully.

Before you eat, explore this food with your sense of smell. What do you notice?

Now, begin eating. No matter how small the bite of food you have, take at least two bites to finish it. Take your first bite. Please chew *very* slowly, noticing the actual sensory experience of chewing and tasting. Remember, you don't need to think about your food to experience it. You might want to close your eyes for a moment to focus on the sensations of chewing and tasting, before continuing.

Notice the texture of the food, the way it feels in your mouth. Notice if the intensity of its flavor changes, moment to moment. Take about 20 more seconds to *very slowly* finish this first bite of food, being aware of the simple sensations of chewing and tasting.

It isn't always necessary to eat slowly in order to eat with mindfulness. But it's helpful at first to slow down, in order to be as mindful as you can.

Now, please take your second and last bite. As before, chew very slowly, while paying close attention to the actual *sensory* experience of eating: the sensations and movements of chewing, the flavor of the food as it changes, and the sensations of swallowing. Just pay attention, moment by moment.

Source: www.MindfulnessDiet.com.

Using a mindfulness eating exercise on a regular basis is only one part of a mindfulness approach to your diet. The liberating power of mindfulness takes deeper effect when you also begin to pay mindful attention to your thoughts and feelings about food, and to the bodily sensations that you are feeling as you eat. It is important to become aware of cues of physical hunger, fullness and satisfaction to decide what, when and how much to eat. Mindfulness (awareness) is the foundation that many people have been missing for overcoming food cravings, addictive eating, binge eating, emotional eating and stress eating.

COLON HYDROTHERAPY

Colon hydrotherapy, sometimes known as colonic irrigation, involves a gentle wash out of the colon, using warm water to remove waste matter, rehydrate and exercise the bowel. Waste material in the colon is flushed out using water squirted through a tube inserted into the rectum while the person lies on their side. The certified colon hydrotherapist controls the pressure and temperature of the water, and the entire procedure usually takes about 45 minutes. Approximately 60 litres of water may be used for the procedure, and some colonic hydrotherapists add herbal infusions to the water first. Massage is also applied to the abdomen by the therapist to ensure an effective cleanse. The combination of massage and water flushing deeply cleanses the colon and releases gas pockets and compacted feces, relieving abdominal bloating and pressure on the lower back, bladder, ovaries/prostate and diaphragm.

History of colon hydrotherapy

Colon hydrotherapy was first practiced by the Egyptians as described in the Ebers Papyrus, the book of medical knowledge of the Egyptians of the 16th century BCE. In ancient times, the practice of cleansing the colon was administered in a river using a hollow reed to induce water flow into the rectum. Colon hydrotherapy became commonly used among Europeans to help with maintenance and promotion of overall health. Enemas, another name for the injection of liquid into the rectum through the anus for cleansing, were frequently used for abatement of fever, anxiety and illness.

At the beginning of the 20th century, the first present day colonic equipment was developed that allowed for a more extensive cleansing of the colon. At that time, Dr John Harvey Kellogg recommended colon hydrotherapy for many ailments, including those of the bile and liver as well as for surgical shock and cholera. He reported in the 1917 *Journal of American Medicine* that in the treatment of 40,000 cases of gastrointestinal disease, he had used surgery in only 20 cases. The others were improved by cleansing of the bowel, improved diet and exercise. However, at that time colonic hydrotherapy was sometimes administered by unskilled and poorly trained individuals, which proved to be detrimental to the support of the general population and the medical profession.

Unfortunately, that disdain is still prevalent among the medical community today even though methods of practice have improved tremendously. Therapist training is now standardized through accrediting associations, such as the International Association for Colon Hydrotherapy (I-ACT) and the National Board for Colon Hydrotherapy (NBCHT) which evaluate the competency of colon hydrotherapy practitioners. One reason for skepticism among scientists and physicians is the sparsity of scientific evidence for the benefits of colon hydrotherapy. However, colon hydrotherapy remains very popular, especially in the UK.

How colon hydrotherapy works and who can benefit

Colon hydrotherapy stimulates the vagus system by temporarily expanding the colon as occurs during peristalsis, activating the stretch receptors in the colonic walls. This causes release of serotonin (5-HT) from the enterochromaffin cells (EC) in the inner surface of the large intestine which stimulates afferent sensory neurons in the mucosa (Figure 6.7).

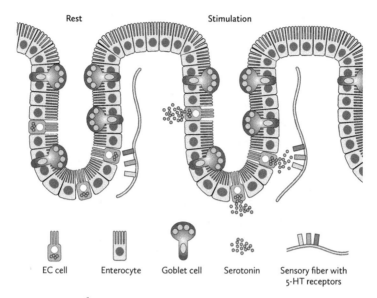

FIGURE 6.7 ENTEROCHROMAFFIN CELLS RELEASING
SEROTONIN IN INTESTINAL MUCOSA.
*Source: Adapted from Mawe GM and Hoffman JM, 2013. Serotonin signalling in
the gut: functions, dysfunctions and therapeutic targets. Nat Rev Gastroenterol
Hepatol. 10(8): 473–486; Figure 1. doi: 10.1038/nrgastro.2013.105.*

These neurons transmit the signal to the nodose ganglion and then to the NTS
which then signals to the dorsal vagal complex to generate peristaltic activity.
The NTS also projects the vagal sensory information regarding gastric distension
to the medulla and amygdala in the limbic system. The increase in vagal tone
indicates to the amygdala that you are in the "rest and digest" state as if you had
just eaten a meal. In this way, colonic treatments are thought to help improve
mental outlook and provide an overall sense of well-being. So, people who have
problems with generalized anxiety could find colon hydrotherapy beneficial,
especially when it is combined with massage and breathing exercises.

The function of peristalsis within the colon is to mix, store and slow the
transportation of intestinal contents so that water from undigested food can be
absorbed into the bloodstream and feces can be evacuated through the rectum
and anus. While peristaltic waves in the small intestine are frequent, those within
the colon occur approximately two to four times per day and are most powerful
in the hour following a meal. In some people, peristalsis is occasionally inhibited,
resulting in constipation and decreased immune function since the intestine is
an important site for local immunity. For that reason, colon hydrotherapy may
improve colon and immune functions in people with constipation. There is some
scientific evidence for improved immune function after colon hydrotherapy.

Colonic irrigation has been shown to increase migration of certain immune cells (lymphocytes) from the gut tissue to the circulation (Uchiyama-Tanaka 2009) so they are available to fight invaders.

Another use of colon hydrotherapy is as a preparation for medical procedures such as a colonoscopy. Some people find this preferable to the traditional method of bowel preparation that involves dietary changes for several days, a liquid diet on the day prior to the colonoscopy and drinking large volumes of unpleasant tasting laxative (Teich *et al.* 2022). According to an excellent review article (Bazzocchi and Giuberti 2017), some controlled studies have appeared comparing the effect of colonic irrigation with conventional treatment approaches for constipation and fecal incontinence. Beyond a shadow of a doubt, they do provide enough data to assert that colonic irrigation is an effective treatment for defecation disorders that have resisted other treatments.

Some complementary and alternative medicine practitioners offer colon cleansing for other purposes, such as detoxification. They believe that toxins from the gastrointestinal tract can cause a variety of health problems, such as arthritis and high blood pressure, and that colon cleansing improves health by removing toxins. However, this theory is controversial. For example, Mayo Clinic Consumer Health and the researcher Francis Seow-Choen (2009) state emphatically that colon hydrotherapy is not necessary for this purpose because the digestive system and bowel already eliminate waste material and bacteria from the body.

Although colon hydrotherapy is safe if performed by a trained, certified colon hydrotherapist (certified by an established institution, such as the National Board for Colon Hydrotherapy or International Association for Colon Hydrotherapy), it is best to avoid colonics if you suffer from certain conditions such as severe kidney or heart disease, or severe hemorrhoids, have recently had abdominal surgery or have an active case of inflammatory bowel disease, such as Crohn's. Your hydrotherapist will determine the suitability of the treatment beforehand.

To summarize, there is scientific evidence that colon hydrotherapy improves bowel function in those whose function is compromised (without active inflammation) and provides the added advantage of stimulating the vagus nerve to increase relaxation, improve mood and outlook, and enhance immune function. The following case study provides further evidence for these benefits in this population in terms of colon hydrotherapy practice in the real world, especially when combined with massage and focus on breathing. However, people without impaired bowel function who wish to engage their vagal nerves may prefer to use other less invasive techniques.

CASE STUDY: Using colon hydrotherapy to tone your vagus and improve your life

Sheila Shea, MA, LMT, NBCHT Certified in Colon Hydrotherapy, Certified GAPS™ Practitioner, Intestinal Heath Institute (intestines@sheilashea.com)

Life before colon hydrotherapy

At 7 years old, SKP entered a hospital emergency room with a bowel blockage (fecal impaction). A nurse removed her impaction by hand. When SKP got home, her bowels emptied prolifically. The nurse gave her mother instructions: prune juice and a sitz bath daily. The doctor said she was completely cleaned out. Not true. She was constipated up to the 7-year-old incident, and that constipation has continued into adulthood. SKP's mother worked away from home during the day and was not aware of her daughter's severe constipation.

> Sometimes I feel I am going to die if I don't poop. Sometimes it can be a whole month. I was taking laxatives every night and they weren't working. You can get colon cancer. I don't want colon cancer. I always feel sluggish. I want to come back to life. I work hard, and sometimes I feel ashamed of myself. I'm tired after work; so, often I didn't have the energy to do things with my kids the way I wanted. [SKP's three children are now 28, 25 and 21 years old.]
>
> Sometimes I feel depression, a lack of energy, and overwhelmed. I lie down in bed after work. I don't clean house. My two dogs are sick. I get depressed cleaning up after them. I am depressed about my life being out of control. I wait until the last minute to do things. I procrastinate, wake up in a panic, overwhelmed.

SKP has experienced constipation, stomach pain and bloating since infancy. She was not breast-fed. She would be described as the crying, colicky baby. As a child, her stool was often covered in mucus. She works in a quiet office, sees many people one-on-one, and is in constant fear of releasing gas. SKP shares her feelings about her intestinal stress. It sounds dire. People with continuous daily constipation, abdominal pain and bloat suffer significant reduction in their quality of life. She was apprehensive about making an initial appointment.

The office setting

My colon hydrotherapy room is peaceful and beautiful. I am fortunate to have large, sliding windows on the second floor overlooking the Santa Catalina Mountain range in Tucson, Arizona (Figure 6.8A). The ceiling is a faux painting of clouds floating through the sky. The colors in the room are mainly blue and white. I have a large reproduction on papyrus of the goddess of the sky, Nut, who swallows the sun at night and births the sun in the morning (Figure 6.8B). The various tools I use on the abdomen during the hydrotherapy session are a vibrator, hot rocks, New Zealand pine belly ball, a three-pronged shiatsu device, a Chi Nei Tsang wooden tummy tool, and a dog tennis ball, plus my hands. I provide mellow background music. Occasionally, incense and essential oils are used.

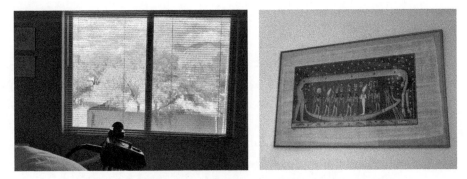

FIGURE 6.8 SHEILA SHEA'S OFFICE. (A) MOUNTAIN VIEW.
(B) CEILING AND PICTURE OF GODDESS OF THE SKY.

SKP came to me initially in 2010 and then returned in 2020. She has been consistent with colon hydrotherapy since then, coming in weekly or every two weeks. She uses various intestinal aids, such as herbal laxatives, magnesium citrate, Dulcolax, stool softeners and charcoal to prepare for the session. She had a straining pattern she has now replaced with breathing. She holds tension in her gut. Her abdomen is usually bloated when she comes in. During the session, her intestinal muscles relax and allow the activation and release of waste. SKP can release the gas and stool, and she feels lighter. Her original discomfort in her abdomen turns into comfort after she can eliminate.

SKP initially came in for her colonic after work on Saturdays. She has changed her schedule because of the difficulty in eliminating and being at work. She now takes the Saturday off, prepares the night before and is free to relax and eliminate in the morning. She then comes in at 2pm in the afternoon for her hydrotherapy. That way, she has a more relaxed and excellent colonic. We use various positions, rotating left side and back positions during the session and using the massage tools. She is prepared, relaxed and can focus on her breath.

Overall, she has progressed to a better, more relaxed way to support her elimination. She has developed a better plan to eliminate and calm her nervous system. Gone are the frenetic days of rushing from work to the colon hydrotherapy session. The whole plan is to make the experience more mindful and restful to the person. To bring down the high-state rush.

The breathing

The more the diaphragm moves, the more stimulation it provides to the vagus nerve, which is why deep breathing is by itself an effective way to improve vagal tone. The person on the table focuses on his/her breath. Before the colon hydrotherapy session, I coach my client on deeper, slower breathing, which includes coherent breathing or heart rate variability, pelvic floor breathing, and yoga breathing, filling the vase from the bottom. The breath is drawn deep into the abdomen. Stimulating the vagus nerve means the person's parasympathetic nervous system opens up and allows the person to relax and release.

Colon hydrotherapy and abdominal massage

Colon hydrotherapy is one of the techniques that helps patients become more self-aware, peaceful and clear-headed as they engage their ventral vagal complex. The vagus nerve connects your gut and brain. Engaging the vagus in colon hydrotherapy activates the parasympathetic nervous system, bringing about relaxation.

Colon hydrotherapy is a gentle, purified-water cleansing of the large intestine, using FDA-approved equipment. The patient rests on a massage table and is connected to the equipment, using disposable tubing and speculum, which have pressure and temperature facility. Warm water and slow inflow allow for the relaxation of the large intestine. The colon hydrotherapy hydrates the system, activates peristalsis and allows waste removal. The warmth of the water, the inflows and outflows at a slow and rhythmic rate and the use of abdominal massage all help the patient rest and relax. As slight pressure builds up in the colon, the water is released. Water and intestinal content flow out through an illuminated glass viewing tube. During the outflows, I massage the abdominal area. The inflows and outflows of water are repeated during the hour-long treatment.

I begin the process in Left Sims position. The patient lies on their left side, head on the pillows, and looks out over the beautiful mountain range. The Left Sims insertion position is a good gas-relieving pose, so we maintain that position for several inflows and outflows to check for gas. Gas is a serious problem, and activating its release allows the person to feel greatly relieved.

The gases may be toxic, and their elimination gives the nervous system a healthier environment. We then rotate to their back where I begin using my massage tools and hands. The patient continues to experience the activation and elimination of gas and waste through the massage and inflows and out-flows of warm water.

Key components of a session:

- Breath.
- Water inflows and outflows that are slow and temperature-controlled.
- Abdominal massage.
- Tools.

Changes I notice after a session indicating that SKP is in a better place
After a session, SKP is less bloated. During the session, she can see waste leaving through a glass viewing tube. She derives satisfaction seeing what is eliminated. She feels emotionally good, like hitting the restart button. She eats a cleaner diet and is motivated to maintain better lifestyle practices. The apprehension she has when she arrives is over. She has an expression of gratitude.

> The night before colonics I take stool softeners, bisacodyl and some magne-sium citrate in water. This usually causes me to go to the bathroom the next morning. I schedule my colonic in the afternoon so the procedure can get even more waste out. After my colonic, I feel relieved that I have succeeded in cleansing my body. My stomach is flatter without the painful bloating I usually have. I feel refreshed and renewed. I am always motivated to eat healthier and not put bad food back into my body. It's like the reset button has been activated. I am always in a good mood after my colonic.

Her posture improves from an initial slump in the lobby to a lovely, straight alignment after she dresses and stands. The strained look of her face is dimin-ished as the muscles of her face soften. She looks brighter as she lifts her chin and smiles after her sessions. Her smile widens. Sometimes she begins laughing and telling me a story.

She is more highly motivated to continue to improve her nutritional pro-gram and create more efficient, relaxed practice around her elimination, such as the taking the day off for the colonic and reducing the rushing from job to colonic. She occasionally takes notes from suggestions or verbal exchanges we have before and/or after the sessions. Better planning and execution of the elimination plan allow for more inner peace and calm. SKP is clearer now what she needs to do to for better and more peaceful elimination. Her words are more positive. Not as drastic and negative as when she first came in. Gone are the days of "I'm gonna die if I don't poop." She loves the little insights on health and lifestyle practice she picks up during our sessions. They excite her. She is an avid student and learner. Her inquisitiveness into her health practices and her excitement about life and how to feel better are palpable.

DAMAGE TO VAGUS NERVE AND IMPAIRED GASTRIC EMPTYING (GASTROPARESIS)

A fully functioning vagus nerve is essential for digestion. If the vagus nerve is damaged, then movement of the gut, or peristalsis, as well as the secretion of digestive enzymes, hormones and mucus are impaired. A case in point is *gastroparesis*, which means partial paralysis of the stomach. This occurs when peristalsis is inhibited such that food moves only very slowly into the intestines from the stomach. This vagal nerve damage can result from diabetes, viral infections, abdominal surgery and scleroderma. Symptoms of gastroparesis are gastroesophageal reflux (backing up of stomach contents into esophagus), vomiting of undigested food, feeling full quickly when eating, chronic abdominal pain, poor appetite and weight loss, and poor blood sugar control.

Common treatments include drugs to induce stomach contraction (which can cause diarrhea), surgical implantation of an electrical stimulator to control vomiting, and gastric bypass surgery which severely limits food intake. In some cases, gastroparesis can be successfully treated much less invasively by stimulating the vagus nerve. In a pilot study (Gottfried-Blackmore *et al.* 2019), 15 patients with gastroparesis used a hand-held, battery-powered electrical stimulator to stimulate the vagus nerve on either side of the neck twice a day for two minutes for a minimum of four weeks. On average, gastric emptying time was reduced from 155 minutes to 129 minutes. These results are promising and follow-up placebo-controlled studies with larger numbers of participants are warranted. Currently, there are several clinical trials in progress.

As described in Chapter 2, another way to stimulate the vagus nerve is by applying acupuncture to the ear. Other acupoints used to access the vagus nerve are PC6 (inside of wrist) and ST36 (on shin one inch from anterior edge of tibia).

There have been a small number of scientific studies to determine whether acupuncture improves symptoms of gastroparesis. Kim *et al.* (2018) reviewed 32 of the published studies that were randomized and placebo-controlled, and concluded:

> There is very low-certainty evidence for a short-term benefit with acupuncture alone or acupuncture combined with gastrokinetic drugs compared with the drug alone, in terms of the proportion of people who experienced improvement in diabetic gastroparesis.

However, in a more recent study (Xuefen *et al.* 2020), 99 patients with gastroparesis were divided into three groups who received acupuncture at different acupuncture points depending on their grouping, for 30 minutes a day for five days during a course of treatment. Three courses of treatment were provided, each separated by two days. In group one, acupuncture points were CV12 (upper abdomen) and ST36; in group two, they were PC6 and ST36; in group three, they were nonacupoint and ST36. The gastroparesis symptom score and the gastric emptying rate were compared before and after treatment for each group. The gastroparesis scores of each group after treatment and at follow-up were significantly lower than those before treatment, and the reduction in the group that received acupuncture at points CV12 and ST36 was the greatest. All three groups showed a significant decrease in gastric emptying time.

A successful case study in which auricular acupuncture was used, as well as acupuncture at other points including PC6 and ST36, for a person with gastroparesis is presented below.

CASE STUDY: Treating gastroparesis with acupuncture
Y. Clare Zhang, PhD, MAcOM, Lac, Practitioner of Integrative Oriental Medicine, Licensed Acupuncturist (y_clare_zhang@hotmail.com)

History and diagnosis
A 56-year-old female patient sought acupuncture in 2014. Her chief complaint was gastroparesis in which the stomach cannot empty itself of food in the normal fashion, which was diagnosed by two gastroenterologists. Her symptoms developed a few days following cholecystectomy (removal of the gallbladder) 13 years prior. The initial symptoms were severe vomiting, constant nausea, frequent diarrhea, weight loss and fatigue. By the time she saw me, some initial symptoms such as vomiting, diarrhea and weight loss had resolved, but others

remained. Her presenting symptoms were constant nausea, fatigue, anxiety, bloating and fullness after a few bites, alternating constipation and diarrhea, and periodic severe upper abdominal pain (i.e., sharp pain behind the sternum).

The patient had tried a number of conventional and alternative medicine approaches with mixed results. Reglan (generic name: metoclopramide), a dopamine antagonist and prokinetic agent, reduced her nausea but caused side effects so serious that she had to discontinue. Improving diet by avoiding processed foods and eating more organic foods alleviated diarrhea. Chiropractic adjustment was very helpful in relieving nausea and esophageal pain for four years, but not any more. Medical marijuana also helped mitigate nausea, and she used it as needed.

Gastroparesis occurs when the vagal nerve is damaged or stops working (Cedars Sinai 2023). Gastroparesis is relatively common following gallbladder surgery. It has been reported that 36–39 percent of gastroparesis patients underwent a prior cholecystectomy (Parkman *et al.* 2013; Deeb *et al.* 2001). One study identified that 8 percent of patients with idiopathic gastroparesis (of unknown cause) had onset of symptoms immediately after cholecystectomy (Soykan *et al.* 1998). It was postulated that vagal nerve damage occurred during the abdominal exploration and removal of the gallbladder.

Based on the fact that gastroparesis symptoms developed shortly after the patient's cholecystectomy, it is highly possible that her vagal nerve was damaged during the surgical procedure. Therefore, I not only designed the acupuncture protocol on the principle of traditional Chinese medicine, but also incorporated the points known to activate the vagal nerve.

Treatments

- Acupuncture: PC6, SP4, ST36, LI10, Ren12, ST25, Ren4.
- Cupping: (in Chinese medicine) a therapy in which heated glass cups are applied to the skin along the meridians of the body, creating suction as a way of stimulating the flow of energy. Gentle moving cupping on the upper back with a focus on T5–T8 vertebrae.
- Auricular acupuncture: Point Zero, Shen Men, San Jiao (aka Triple Burner), Endocrine, Digestive Subcortex, Stomach, Cardia, Liver, Gallbladder. This is done with acupuncture needles or ear seeds which are small seeds used to stimulate pressure points in the ear. I taught the patient to apply ear seeds for herself, so she can extend the therapeutic results.

- Acupressure: PC6 and SP4. I recommended Sea Bands in her first appointment. Sea Bands are a pair of acupressure wrist bands clinically proven to relieve nausea, morning sickness and motion sickness. They have buttons applying constant pressure to the acupuncture point PC6. They are so helpful for her nausea that she has worn them since then. SP4 is a fantastic point for severe upper abdominal pain. This point is located on the feet. When she has sharp pain behind the sternum, she would ask her husband to rub SP4, which would give her immediate relief without fail.
- Herbs and supplements: Huo Xiang Zheng Qi Pian is a Chinese herbal medicine. It is a great remedy for indigestion, bloating, fullness, stomach flu and abdominal pain. Gamma oryzanol is a natural supplement extracted from rice bran oil. Low-dose gamma oryzanol 10–15mg, 2–3 times a day, can stimulate vagal nerve. High-dose gamma oryzanol, 60–100mg, three times a day, can suppress vagal nerve.

Results

Each acupuncture treatment offers the patient complete relief of all her gastroparesis symptoms for one week. She extends the effects longer with acupressure, ear seed application and herbal supplements. She has been very happy with the results.

Mechanisms

Many studies have demonstrated vagal nerve activation as an important mechanism underlying the therapeutic effects of acupuncture in cardiovascular, digestive, psycho-emotional and pain conditions. PC6 is a point on the forearm which, when stimulated, can increase gastric motility and decrease heart rate and blood pressure (Lu et al. 2019; Li et al. 2010). These effects are mainly mediated by stimulation of vagal nerve activity (Lu et al. 2019) and inhibition of sympathetic activity (Li et al. 2010). A 2021 study published in Nature demonstrated that electroacupuncture stimulation of the hindlimb ST36 acupuncture point in mice can activate hindbrain efferent vagal neurons and release catecholamine from adrenal glands, thereby driving the vagal-adrenal anti-inflammatory pathway (Liu et al. 2021).

Besides acupuncture points on the body, many auricular points are particularly powerful in modulating the nervous system. For instance, Shen Men and Point Zero can induce parasympathetic activation and minimize the change in postoperative heart rate variability (Arai et al. 2013).

The sympathetic nerves regulating the stomach originate from the thoracic spine, mainly T5–T8. I use cupping to relax sympathetic nerves in this area. Cupping is a great myofascial treatment that opens up fascia, relaxes muscles and improves blood circulation and lymphatic drainage. Cupping on the thoracic spine helps decrease pressure and irritation to the nerves arising from these segments.

In summary, scientific evidence for the efficacy of acupuncture to treat gastroparesis is in its infancy, but initial results look promising.

GUT BACTERIA: THE MICROBIOME

How gut bacteria communicate with the brain

The microbiome is the collection of bacteria, fungi, viruses, and their genes, that naturally live on the inner surface of the gut. The colon microbiome is one of the most populated microbial habitats found on Earth. Dominant gut microbial phyla are Firmicutes, Bacteroidetes, Actinobacteria, Proteobacteria, Fusobacteria, and Verrucomicrobia. Firmicutes and Bacteroidetes represent 90% of gut microbiota.

Changes in the microbiome are detected by peripheral nerves in the intestinal mucosa which transmit this information to the limbic system directly via activation of vagal afferent nerves, or indirectly by stimulating enteroendocrine cells in the gut to release hormones and neurotransmitters that then activate vagal afferent nerves. In addition to their role in the regulation of intestinal functions such as motility, secretion and activation of immune responses, the gut microbiome also influences higher neural functions, including mood as depicted in Figure 6.2.

Microbiologist Mark Lyte proposed a neurochemical "delivery system" by which gut bacteria, such as probiotics, can send messages to the brain (Lyte 2011). Gut bacteria produce and respond to the same neurochemicals, such as GABA, serotonin, norepinephrine, dopamine, acetylcholine and melatonin, that the brain uses to regulate mood and cognition. Such neurochemicals may allow the brain to augment its responses to the signals it receives from the troops of bacteria in the gut.

The microbiome and diet

The signals that the microbiome sends to the brain through the vagus nerve may be altered by diet, especially probiotics. Probiotics are live bacteria and yeasts that, when eaten in adequate amounts, are beneficial to human health. They are usually added to yoghurt or taken as food supplements. Researchers showed that eating yoghurt twice daily can help treat depression and that the probiotics in the yoghurt affect areas of the brain related to emotions and pain (Tillisch *et al.* 2013). Although the biological mechanisms behind these changes are unclear, it is known that gut bacteria send signals to the brain that can change over time depending on diet.

Another study found that a 30-day course of probiotic bacteria (a mix of *Lactobacillus helveticus* and *Bifidobacteria longum*) led to decreased anxiety and depression in healthy human volunteers (Messaoudi *et al.* 2011). Lower levels of *Bifidobacteria* and *Lactobacillus* have been found in people with depression, compared with those without (Aizawa *et al.* 2016). Scientists hope that a probiotic therapy may one day be available for conditions including anxiety, depression and even autism and Alzheimer's disease, but further investigations are needed.

Key messages from an excellent review of the gut microbiota in nutrition and health (Valdez *et al.* 2018) are shown in Box 6.2.

BOX 6.2 REVIEW OF GUT MICROBIOTA

- Gut microbiota influences many areas of human health from innate immunity to appetite and energy metabolism.
- Targeting the gut microbiome, with probiotics or dietary fiber, benefits human health and could potentially reduce obesity.
- Drugs, food ingredients, antibiotics and pesticides could all have adverse effects on the gut microbiota.
- Microbiota should be considered a key aspect in nutrition; the medical community should adapt their education and public health messages.
- Fiber consumption is associated with beneficial effects in several contexts.

Emotions affect gut microbiota: a two-way street

Just as gut bacteria affect the brain, the brain can also exert profound influences on the gut microbiome, with feedback effects on behavior. Numerous studies have shown that psychological stress suppresses beneficial bacteria. In a 2004 study in the *Journal of Pediatric Gastroenterology and Nutrition*, Bailey *et al.* found that infant monkeys whose mothers had been startled by loud noises during pregnancy had fewer *Lactobacilli* and *Bifidobacteria* (Bailey *et al.* 2004). The results also extend to humans. In 2008, Simon Knowles and colleagues found that during exam week, university students' stool samples contained fewer *Lactobacilli* than they had during the less stressful first few days of the semester (Knowles *et al.* 2008).

In summary, regardless of whether or not you suffer from depression, eating yoghurt with added probiotics and fermented foods such as sauerkraut and kim-chi (both fermented vegetable mixes) that are rich in beneficial bacteria helps to maintain equilibrium in the gut. In addition, eating a wide variety of vegetables and fruits can help to provide prebiotic fibers for bacteria to break down, which provides them with the essential fuel they need to maintain themselves and create the metabolites that positively influence brain function.

Although the research is still in its initial stages, it appears that eating such foods will induce the vagus nerve to send signals from the gut to the brain, to benefit your emotional health. In addition, by using one of the methods described in this book to activate your vagus nerve, you will culture the growth of more diverse and beneficial bacteria in your gut. The following case study describes successful use of dietary changes to improve vagal function as evidenced by a restoration of healthy digestion and a calm state of mind.

> The doctor of the future will no longer treat the human frame with drugs, but rather will cure and prevent disease with nutrition. (Thomas Edison, inventor and businessman)

CASE STUDY: Effects of diet on the microbiome

Sheila Shea, MA, LMT, NBCHT Certified in Colon Hydrotherapy, Certified GAPS™ Practitioner, Intestinal Heath Institute (intestines@sheilashea.com)

Much of the information about the intestinal mucosal environment is sent to the brain via the vagus nerve, and the vagus nerve also mediates effects of dietary changes on the mucosa and on the emotions.

In 2019, RAR was up and down with a nutritional protocol called Gut and Psychology Syndrome diet (GAPS). He had practiced it for six weeks two different times. He was on and off the GAPS diet because he could not control his sugar cravings. The sugar tiger had him by the tail! He felt more tired, had low energy, had some improvement, and abandoned it again. He continued the Wise Traditions, Weston A Price Foundation (WAPF) protocol authored by Sally Fallon, with fermented foods including fermenting complex carbohydrate grains, and felt some improvement. He continually craved sugars and found the fermentation of grains kept him from consuming junk sugars. I saw him that year. An incidence of blood in his stool got his attention, and he wanted more insight and help to support his gut using GAPS.

RAR came to me on December 6, 2019, shortly after his bout with rectal bleeding. On his first visit, he was very frustrated about his rectal bleeding and sugar addiction. He described himself as anxious, irritable and restless, with panic attacks while eliminating. RAR appeared nervous, slightly pale, thin and angular. His weight dropped to 130 pounds from 150. On any given day, he had anywhere from 6 to 20 diarrhea eliminations, many with mucus. He could not socialize with this scenario. He realized he was in a wasting condition. Edgy and agitated, he wanted answers.

His muscles were tight and he had a contracted appearance. He suffered from insomnia. He slumped in his chair. He said he was losing electrolytes from all the diarrhea, and was weak and at his wit's end. He described night terrors, a sense of obsessive-compulsive disorder with his work and a craving for starch, fructose and glucose. He was tired of his ups and downs with sugar. He had been on and off the GAPS diet and couldn't get consistency with healthy carbohydrates. With other symptoms of bad breath and foul-smelling gas, he speculated infection and microbiome imbalance.

Spoiler alert! Development of rectal cancer

In the fall of 2000, RAR began working for himself. He believed his behavior from 2010 to 2018 and the associated stress led to his diagnosis of rectal cancer in 2020. He wanted to earn more so that he could retire. His sleep was irregular. His diet declined. He provoked his sympathetic nervous system rather than stroking his parasympathetic nervous system. Poor vagus! The early symptoms in 2016–2017 were minor constipation and diarrhea. By 2017, these symptoms settled down and went away. However, in the middle 2018, he had blood in his stool. He found Campbell-McBride and the GAPS protocol and began it immediately. These protocols give recognition to the importance of the microbiome, the world of bacteria, fungi and virus that inhabit the gut and our whole body. These protocols include fermented foods that support the growth of the healthy microbes in the gut and reduce the negative.

After reading and practicing GAPS in 2018, RAR realized the importance of gut health and that our microbiome vastly outnumbers our human cells. Certain nutritional protocols, the Specific Carbohydrate Diet, GAPS and WAPF have documented healing from inflammatory bowel disease (IBD) and irritable bowel syndrome through reducing or eliminating foods that feed the wrong microbial population, and then feeding the healthy microorganisms. Chronic diarrhea falls under the umbrella of IBD. RAR has a history of chronic diarrhea and displayed symptoms of ulcerative colitis, specifically diarrhea and bloody diarrhea. Chronic inflammation in the bowel and elsewhere can lead to various cancers – in his case, rectal cancer. The diet is a major healing influence on the microbiome. Cancer is another condition in which the person suffers from a serious imbalance in their microbiome.

Diagnosis and treatment

One evening in March 2020, he experienced serious bleeding in the afternoon. He could not control the bleeding and later that evening went to the emergency room and spent three days in the hospital. He had a tumor growth in his rectum and was diagnosed with Stage 3 rectal cancer. It had not metastasized. "When I first got the cancer diagnosis I was not scared. Somehow, I felt something positive might come out of it."

During April and May 2020, he opted for conventional chemotherapy and radiation treatment. In August 2020, after the colorectal cancer diagnosis, RAR began seeing a naturopathic medical doctor (NMD) specializing in oncology. The NMD gave RAR vitamin C IV drips and some supplements. After seeing what he had taken and was prescribed, the NMD told RAR, "This stuff is hard on the gut lining. It could take several years to restore it."

Chemicals and radiation are damaging to the gut lining, the fragile epithelial cells that line our gastrointestinal tract. These substances clearly imbalance our microbiome balance and health. The degradation of the gut wall allows substances into the circulatory system for distribution to the body. The reverse is true. The good microbes send good messages to the brain that allow for neurological healing and vagal stimulation. For example, oxytocin is produced in the brain through positive microbes such as *Lactobacillus reuteri* according to studies by William Davis, MD, in his 2022 book, *Super Gut*.

During the four weeks of chemotherapy, RAR had cramping in his intestines. Computerized tomography scans showed the tumor shrinking. He felt encouraged that he was going in the right direction. In the fourth week of radiation, the scans showed a build-up of stool in the bowel. He took Senokot and cleared the impactions in his large intestines. On the fifth week, he developed severe diarrhea and needed disposable underwear. After the fifth week of chemotherapy, the diarrhea subsided. The chemotherapy clearly affected his microbiome adversely, causing the diarrhea; one of RAR's main issues is diarrhea and urgent stool elimination. In April 2021, MRI and CT scans showed a reduction of the tumor to Stage 1, a minor mass. His circulating tumor cells test was negative. A final December 2021 MRI showed nothing left but scar tissue. What a relief! His work with diet and supplements had paid off.

Diet and supplements during and after chemotherapy and radiation

RAR was slowly progressing on the WAPF protocol before his cancer diagnosis. Chemotherapy and radiation changed his diet and appetite. The most noticeable change was in his desire for and consumption of junk food, along with the WAPF protocol. After the chemotherapy and radiation, he lost the desire for the junk food, his appetite normalized and he hit the WAPF protocol even harder. The tissue burning from radiation and the side effects of chemotherapy went away. Other effects, like spots before his eyes and an irregular heartbeat, were gone.

During cancer treatment, milk was the "only appetizing thing, plus the junk." Most of his diet was eggs, a quart of raw milk daily, plus junk food. Raw milk continues to be a staple in his diet. The glutathione from raw milk protein allows "the rapid multiplication of immune-enhancing white blood cells and is an antioxidant and detoxifier of the cell." The milk provides the needed support of his immune system while allowing the good microbes to affect his vagus nerve positively. The raw milk also contains beneficial microorganisms that help digestion of the milk proteins naturally.

After being free of rectal cancer, he discontinued the vitamin C infusions and supplements A, D and K2 previously suggested by his NMD. He uses a fermented cod liver oil and concentrated butter oil blend from Green Pasture. This blend of oils is nutrient-rich and full of healthy fats to boost brain and nervous system support. The stimulation and health of the vagus nerve depends upon a healthy supply of appropriate fats. RAR ferments vegetables for his pre- and probiotics and consumes them daily. He begins his day drinking water with a quarter teaspoon of Celtic sea salt and uses it in his culinary practice. The salt provides electrolytes rich in minerals essential for overall bodily functions. His main calories consumed are grains, raw milk and butter. He consumes bone stock for rebuilding of the epithelial cells of the gut. According to the WAPF and GAPS protocols, his grains are fermented and non-GMO. The fermentation of grains makes the food more assimilable and increases the quantity of nutrients. Some Native American corn is heirloom and sourced locally. Eggs, meat and cheese are also a part of his diet.

My job is healing myself and my continued work pays off! I am releasing everything from my awareness that lacks the confidence to achieve this healing for myself. Stay tuned...

Over the years, RAR has plugged away at improving his practice of adding probiotic and fermented foods to his diet and eating organic, nutrient-dense foods. The continued accumulation of positive microbes in his dietary practice has contributed to a healthier microbiome and has allowed the continued healing of his GI tract and stimulation of his vagus nerve. He began exercising again in late 2020. He feels his cardiovascular fitness is better now than before. His weight has stabilized around 150 pounds. He started his retirement in the fall of 2018 and completed it in June of 2021. He is experiencing positive improvements in his gut health although he still experiences minor episodes of urgent elimination. He added *Saccharomyces boulardii*, another potent positive microbe, for his diarrhea and urgent stool. Healing takes time.

His healing of cancer through nutrition led to other levels of inner healing, his emotional and mental bodies. RAR feels a deeper sense of relaxation and continues to work toward internal mental peace. That can be attributed to a greater healing of his overall body and nervous system. He feels that "No matter what is going on around me, I can remain at peace. That is the goal. Whether small or big things upset me, the key is inner peace." He devotes time to quiet inner listening. He recovers from negative reactions more quickly and is better at not judging himself. Through WAPF protocol he is better able to hear intuition and inner guidance. He has an overall sense of better calmness which results from the more peaceful nervous system. Cancer was a strong wakeup call. He moved away from the sympathetic rush world and moved toward a more parasympathetic relaxed state. He moves from his nutrition to his enhanced microbiome, to the vagal finale, inner peace.

Resources
www.westonaprice.org/the-biochemical-magic-of-raw-milk-and-other-raw-foods-glutathione

Davis W, 2022. *Super Gut: A Four-Week Plan to Reprogram Your Microbiome, Restore Health, and Lose Weight.* Paris: Hachette Go.

REFERENCES

Aizawa E, Tsuji H, Asahara T *et al.*, 2016. Possible association of *Bifidobacterium* and *Lactobacillus* in the gut microbiota of patients with major depressive disorder. *J Affect Disord.* 202: 254-7, 2016. doi: 10.1016/j.jad.2016.05.038.

Arai Y, Sakakima Y, Kawanish J *et al.*, 2013. Auricular acupuncture at the "Shenmen" and "Point Zero" points induced parasympathetic activation. *Evid Based Complement Alternat Med.* 2013: 945063.

Bai L, Mesgarzadeh S, Ramesh KS *et al.*, 2019. Genetic identification of vagal sensory neurons that control feeding. *Cell.* 179 (5): 1129, 2019. doi: 10.1016/j.cell.2019.10.031.

Bailey MT, Lubach GR and Coe CL., 2004. Prenatal stress alters bacterial colonization of the gut in infant monkeys. *J Pediatr Gastroenterol Nutr.* 38(4): 414–421. doi: 10.1097/00005176-200404000-00009.

Bays JC, 2009. *Mindful Eating. A Guide to Rediscovering a Healthy and Joyful Relationship with Food.* Shambhala Publications.

Bazzocchi G and Giuberti R, 2017. Irrigation, lavage, colonic hydrotherapy: from beauty center to clinic? *Tech Coloproctol.* 21(1): 1–4. doi: 10.1007/s10151-016-1576-6.

Berthoud HR and Neuhuber WL, 2000. Functional and chemical anatomy of the afferent vagal system. *Auton Neurosci.* 85:1–17. doi: 10.1016/S1566-0702(00)00215-0.

Breit S, Kupferberg A, Rogler G and Hasler G, 2018. Vagus nerve as modulator of the brain-gut axia in psychiatric and inflammatory disorders. *Frontiers in Psychiatry.* www.frontiersin.org/articles/10.3389/fpsyt.2018.00044/full.

Buchanan KL, Rupprecht LE, Kaelberer MM *et al.*, 2022. The preference for sugar over sweetener depends on a gut sensor cell. *Nat Neurosci.* 25: 191–200. doi: 10.1038/s41593-021-00982-7.

Cedars Sinai, 2023. Gastroparesis. Available from: www.cedars-sinai.org/health-library/diseases-and-conditions/g/gastroparesis.html#:~:text=Gastroparesis%20is%20caused%20when%20your,too%20slowly%20or%20stops%20moving.

Deeb F, Lacy B, Yoo H *et al.*, 2001. Gastroparesis: a risk factor for cholecystectomy? *Am J Gastroenterol.* 96(9 Suppl): S51–S52.

Furness JB, 2009. Enteric nervous system. In: Binder MD, Hirokawa N, Windhorst U (Eds). *Encyclopedia of Neuroscience.* Berlin, Heidelberg: Springer; Figure 1. doi: 10.1007/978-3-540-29678-2_3035.

Gottfried-Blackmore A, Adler EP, Fernandez-Becker N *et al.*, 2019. Open-label pilot study: non-invasive vagal nerve stimulation improves symptoms and gastric emptying in patients with idiopathic gastroparesis. *Neurogastroenterol Motil.* 32(4): e13769. doi: 10.1111/nmo.13769.

Herman MA, Cruz MT, Sahlbzada N *et al.*, 2009. GABA signaling in the nucleus tractus solitarius sets the level of activity in dorsal motor nucleus of the vagus cholinergic neurons in the vagovagal circuit. *American Journal of Physiology, Gastrointestinal and Liver Physiology.* 296(1): G101–G111. doi: 10.1152/ajpgi.90504.2008.

Kim KH, Lee MS, Choi TY and Kim TH, 2018. Acupuncture for symptomatic gastroparesis. *Cochrane Database Syst Rev.* 12(12): CD009676. doi: 10.1002/14651858.CD009676.pub2.

Knowles SR, Nelson EA and Palombo EA, 2008. Investigating the role of perceived stress on bacterial flora activity and salivary cortisol secretion: a possible mechanism underlying susceptibility to illness. *Biol Psychol.* 77(2): 132–137. doi: 10.1016/j.biopsycho.2007.09.010.

Li P and Longhurst J, 2010. Neural mechanism of electroacupuncture's hypotensive effects. *Autonomic Neuroscience: Basic and Clinical.* 157: 24–30.

Liu S, Wang Z, Su Y *et al.*, 2021. A neuroanatomical basis for electroacupuncture to drive the vagal-adrenal axis. *Nature.* 598(7882): 641–645.

Lu M, Chen C, Li W *et al.*, 2019. EA at PC6 promotes gastric motility: role of brainstem vagovagal neurocircuits. *Evid Based Complement Alternat Med.* 2019: 7457485.

Lyte M, 2011. Probiotics function mechanistically as delivery vehicles for neuroactive compounds: microbial endocrinology in the design and use of probiotics. *Bioessays.* 33(8): 574–581. doi: 10.1002/bies.201100024.

Messaoudi M, Lalonde R, Violle N *et al.*, 2011. Assessment of psychotropic-like properties of a pro-biotic formulation (*Lactobacillus helveticus* R0052 and *Bifidobacterium longum* R0175) in rats and human subjects. *British Journal of Nutrition.* 105(5): 755-764. doi: 10.1017/S0007114510004319.

Parkman HP, Yates K, Hasler WL *et al.*, 2013. Cholecystectomy and clinical presentations of gastroparesis. *Dig Dis Sci.* 58(4):1062-73.

Prins RD, 2011. The brain-gut interaction: the conversation and the implications. *South African Journal of Clinical Nutrition.* 24 (Sup3): 8–14. doi: 10.1080/16070658.2011.11734373.

Seow-Choen F, 2009. The physiology of colonic hydrotherapy. *Colorectal Disease.* 11: 686–688.

Soykan I, Sivri B, Sarosiek I *et al.*, 1998. Demography, clinical characteristics, psychological and abuse profiles, treatment, and long-term follow-up of patients with gastroparesis. *Dig Dis Sci.* 43: 2398–2404.

Stanhope KL, 2016. Sugar consumption, metabolic disease and obesity: the state of the controversy. *Crit Rev Clin Lab Sci.* 53(1): 52–67. doi: 10.3109/10408363.2015.1084990.

Teich N, Klecker C, Klugmann T and Dietel P, 2022. Bowel preparation prior to colonoscopy with a new colonic irrigation device: results of a prospective observational study. *Endosc Int Open.* 10: E971–E977. doi: 10.1055/a-1858-3728.

Tillisch K, Labus J, Kilpatrick L *et al.*, 2013. Consumption of fermented milk product with pro-biotic modulates brain activity. *Gastroenterology.* 144(7): 1394–1401, 1401.e1-4. doi: 10.1053/j.gastro.2013.02.043.

Uchiyama-Tanaka Y, 2009. Colon irrigation causes lymphocyte movement from gut-associated lymphatic tissues to peripheral blood. *Biomedical Research.* 30(5): 311–314.

Valdez AM, Walter J, Segal E and Spector T, 2018. Role of the gut microbiota in nutrition and health. *BMJ.* doi: 10.1136/bmj.k2179.

Xuefen W, Ping L, Li L *et al.*, 2020. A clinical randomized controlled trial of acupuncture treatment of gastroparesis using different acupoints. *Pain Research and Management.* 2020: 8751958. doi: 10.1155/2020/8751958.

Zhu JX, Zhu XY, Owyang C and Li Y, 2001. Intestinal serotonin acts as a paracrine substance to mediate vagal signal transmission evoked by luminal factors in the rat. *J Physiol.* 530(Pt 3): 431–442. doi: 10.1111/j.1469-7793.2001.0431k.x.

CHAPTER 7

The Limbic System

SOMATIC THERAPY

INTRODUCTION

Somatic therapy is an overall term for therapies that center on the mind-body connection. It relies on the assumption that pent-up trauma becomes "trapped" in the body and can be released using a variety of techniques with the aid of a therapist. The limbic system is important in somatic therapy because it mediates communication between the mind and the body. In this chapter, we will add more detail to our initial description of the limbic system.

We will then move on to the insula, a part of the brain cortex closely connected to the limbic system, which is a major hub for incoming messages from your body about the physical sensations you are feeling. To dispel harmful, stress-related changes to your anatomy and physiology, it is first necessary to acknowledge them and to discover exactly where they are located, how extensive they are and what quality of sensations they evoke. The insula collects that information mainly via the vagus nerve and its cranial branches from viscerosensory pathways emerging from the internal organs, and from somatosensory pathways coming from the skin. The insula then passes the information along to the prefrontal cortex and you consciously perceive your inner state. The process of becoming aware of your bodily sensations is called "interoception." Somatic therapists can help to improve skills of interoception by utilizing the "body scan," a central element of the mindfulness-based stress reduction program first developed by Kabat-Zinn in 1979 (Kabat-Zinn 2003) described later in this chapter.

Next, we will explore the details of how chronic stress manifests itself in the body, including the release of various stress hormones and neurotransmitters and their effects on the limbic system, prefrontal cortex, internal organs and skeletal muscles. Finally, we will describe some of the mind-body techniques used in somatic therapy to detect and release tension, focusing on the role of the vagus nerve and its cranial branches. This section will be illustrated by a case study from a physical therapist.

The idea that stress can become "trapped" in the body is interesting, but this term is not very scientific. I think that this phrase actually refers to the lasting chemical, hormonal, cellular and structural changes that manifest in the body following periods of chronic emotional stress that may be initiated by acute trauma. Trauma can shift the ANS into a state of sympathetic hyperarousal ("fight or flight" response) or, in severe cases, into a parasympathetic freeze response, in which the dorsal vagus nerve is so highly stimulated that profound relaxation occurs such that one becomes immobilized and heart rate drops.

Hyperarousal is associated with an overactive amygdala, and the freeze response (hypoarousal) with an underactive amygdala. As described in Chapter 4, the amygdala is closely connected to all other components of the limbic system as well as the prefrontal cortex, and so its level of activity will influence the release of stress hormones and neurotransmitters, memory recall and cognitive skills. Stress hormones and neurotransmitters affect the immune system, digestive system, glucose metabolism, muscle mass, brain function and the density and complexity of neural connections, so it is not surprising that chronic imbalances in their release have deleterious effects on the mind and body. For this reason, trauma and chronic stress can impair physiological function, memory recall and emotional regulation. In addition, stress causes contraction of skeletal muscle. When muscles are tense, the blood circulation decreases, and lactic acid builds up, causing pain and stiffness. In order to break the cycle of chronic stress, whether it comes from a "fight or flight" or a "dorsal freeze" response, it is necessary to stimulate the ventral vagus complex (Figure 7.1).

As described in the previous chapters of this book, there are multiple ways to stimulate the ventral vagus complex, including techniques related to breath regulation, emotional perception, somatosensory awareness and social engagement. By honing these skills, the activity of the amygdala will restabilize, emotional trauma will dissipate and tension in the body will be released. What underlies all somatic therapies is the belief that the body can manifest mental and emotional unease and can also help heal it.

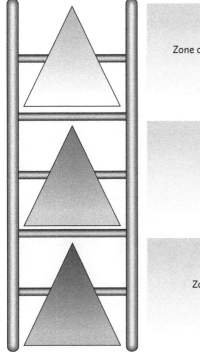

Zone of safety, calmness, relaxed alertness, social engagement
Ventral vagal complex

Zone of agitation, stress, fear, anxiety, aggression
Sympathetic component

Zone of grief, numbness, denial, lack of joy, stuckness
Dorsal vagal complex

FIGURE 7.1 AUTONOMIC LADDER.
Source: Adapted from Deb Dana, LCSW.

COMPONENTS OF THE LIMBIC SYSTEM AND THEIR FUNCTIONS

The limbic system is a group of brain structures organized into a functional unit that is important for the expression of emotional and mood states. Your emotional experience is the combination of stimuli that your brain receives from the external environment and the internal sensations that are transmitted to the brain from bodily organs and systems. As seen in Figure 7.2, there are six groups of inputs to the limbic system, so the limbic system deals with a lot of information.

The inputs to the limbic system most relevant to trauma are sensory input from skeletal muscles via the somatic sensory nerves, which contribute information related to muscle tension, and information from the brain stem and ANS. The brain stem and ANS are important because they are used by the viscero-sensory pathways to convey sensory information from the visceral organs, such as that tight feeling in your stomach. The ANS obtains signals both directly from the nerve endings in the visceral organs, and indirectly from hormones that are released by cells in the visceral organs which then stimulate local nerve endings. This latter route is mediated by the endocrine system.

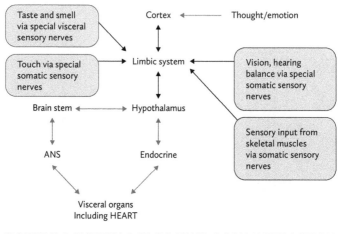

FIGURE 7.2 PHYSIOLOGY OF MIND-BODY INTERACTION.
Note connections to the limbic system.

There are four main components of the limbic system: the thalamus, hypothalamus, hippocampus and the amygdala, as shown in Figure 7.3.

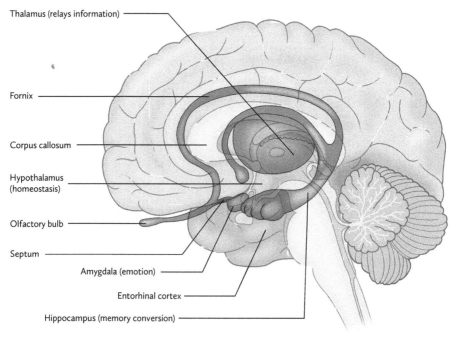

FIGURE 7.3 COMPONENTS OF THE LIMBIC SYSTEM
Source: Adapted from © 2022 Quizlet Inc.

The thalamus is a small, egg-shaped structure central to the brain that sits deep in the brain at the top of the brain stem. It is known as the gateway to the cerebral cortex because it relays motor and sensory information to specific regions in the cortex. Nearly all sensory inputs from other areas of the nervous system pass through the thalamus to the cerebral cortex. Injury to this special structure can lead to loss of senses.

The hypothalamus is a smaller, spherical feature that sits under the front region of the thalamus, on top of the brain stem. It is about the size of an almond. Its major function is to maintain the body's internal balance (homeostasis). To do this, it regulates heart rate and blood pressure, body temperature, thirst (for fluid balance), appetite, sleep cycles, glandular secretions of the stomach and intestines, and production of biochemicals that influence the pituitary gland to release hormones. It is considered to be the link between the ANS and the endocrine system.

The hippocampus consists of a pair of crescent-shaped structures located on each side of the brain. Hippocampus means seahorse in Greek, and each hippocampus looks like a seahorse due to the way it is folded during development. As already described, it is associated with the formation and storage of explicit memories to do with learning and events (declarative memory). Explicit memories are those requiring conscious thought, such as remembering who came to dinner last night, whereas implicit memory is a type of memory that is not usually consciously recalled, such as how to ride a bicycle.

The amygdala consists of a pair of small, almond-shaped structures located toward the bottom of the brain on the left and right sides. The amygdala is related to emotional responses in people, especially fear, anger and hedonistic pleasure seeking. If unregulated, the response of the amygdala can lead to creation of irrational fears or phobias. As mentioned in Chapter 4, the amygdala warns the body of certain stimuli that might threaten its survival. Many sensory inputs are linked to the amygdala to inform it of potential dangers in the environment. Although such inputs are very important, the amygdala also receives information about non-threatening happenings in the surroundings from the sensory cortex in the brain relating to the five senses. So, your state of arousal could also be reduced by what you are experiencing in the environment if it feels safe. The amygdala is closely connected to the hippocampus, and this juxtaposition may be the reason that memories connected with an important emotional event are etched deeply into our consciousness. These connections between the amygdala and the sensory cortex, and the amygdala and the hippocampus are shown in Figure 7.4.

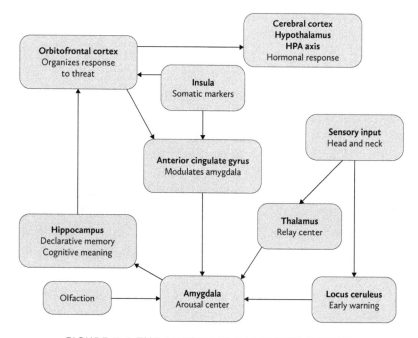

FIGURE 7.4 THE AUTONOMIC NERVOUS SYSTEM.
Source: Figure 3.1: The Limbic Brain, from 8 KEYS TO BRAIN-BODY BALANCE by Robert Scaer. Copyright © 2012 by Robert Scaer, MD. Used by permission of W. W. Norton & Company, Inc.

As we shall learn later in this chapter, somatotherapists often encourage their clients to take notice of objects in the environment to steady their attention and reduce the overwhelming response of their amygdala.

Another important structure that is not technically part of the limbic system, but is closely associated, is the anterior cingulate cortex (ACC), or gyrus. According to information that it receives from the prefrontal cortex and the insula (which senses the internal state of the body), the ACC modulates the activity of the amygdala. As an example, imagine you are walking through the woods, thinking you are alone, and suddenly you hear a branch crack behind you. That information is transmitted from the sensory cortex to the amygdala. As a result, you are startled, and your amygdala becomes highly stimulated. You quickly look behind you and then see the harmless fox that was responsible for the noise. You breathe a sigh of relief. Your ACC has received the information from your prefrontal cortex that the noise was caused by a fox, and the information from your insula that you have released some tension from your body. The ACC feeds that information into the amygdala. As a result, your amygdala quietens down and you consciously experience a sense of relief. To summarize, the ACC helps integrate thinking and feeling using information from the prefrontal cortex and insula. All these responses are illustrated in Figure 7.4.

THE INSULA: RECEIVER OF BODILY SENSATIONS

The insula resides in the cerebral cortex adjacent to the prefrontal cortex. It senses the internal state of the body and is an essential component of the pain matrix, a set of brain areas including the thalamus and ACC, that consistently responds to painful stimuli. The sensations recorded by the insula derive from the following nerve sources:

- Sensory organs in the head send information to the limbic system via special visceral and somatic sensory (afferent) nerves.
- Visceral organs (heart, gut, lungs) send information to the limbic system via visceral sensory (afferent) nerves adjacent to the spinal cord (sympathetic) and in the vagus nerve (parasympathetic; tractus solitarius nerve fibers in the vagus).
- Skeletal muscles send sensory information to the limbic system via somatic sensory (afferent) nerves.

The insula assesses the intensity of gut feelings, muscular aches and contractions, and informs the brain about our state of well-being, or otherwise. As shown in Figure 7.4, the insula also sends information about bodily sensations to the ACC. As we have all observed, feelings that are pleasant are usually associated with tranquility, whereas those that involve pain, tension or discomfort often put us into a state of hypervigilance. These associations between sensations and mood stem from physiology. The extent to which the hypothalamus activates a "fight or flight," or hypervigilance, response depends on the sensory information from the rest of the body, which is provided by the insula. Sensory signals associated with feelings of relaxation instruct the ACC to tone down the amygdala, so the hypothalamus reduces the "fight or flight" response, whereas sensations related to pain and tension will excite the amygdala and increase the "fight or flight" response. This is why the insula and the ACC are very important in somatic therapy.

As will be described later in this chapter, one technique used by somatotherapists to help their clients release tension is to encourage them to pay close attention to sensations within their body and note how the sensations change when they make the conscious decision to release tension. The idea is that if we reduce tension in the body, the valence of our emotions will improve, going from unpleasant to pleasant. As our emotional state improves, this will influence our thoughts. Emotions and thoughts are often aligned in valence (Lagattuta *et al.* 2016), pleasant emotions with positive thoughts.

This technique of influencing emotions and thoughts by means of acknowledging body sensations is known as "bottom-up" processing, and was developed by psychotherapist Peter Levine as part of his program, "Somatic Experiencing." The theory behind somatic experiencing is that post-traumatic stress disorder (PTSD) symptoms are an expression of stress activation. The key to working with the emotions in the bottom-up approach is that while you are feeling emotions, you bring your attention into your body. Are there places of tension? Do you feel hot or cold? Are you breathing quickly or slowly? Are your breaths shallow or deep? As you focus more on your body, your body then has more of a chance to release tension and return to neutral.

POST-TRAUMATIC STORAGE OF TENSION IN THE BODY

Muscle tension

When the body is under a level of constant mental or emotional stress, physical symptoms begin to emerge. The hyperactive status of the amygdala triggers the release of stress hormones such as epinephrine, norepinephrine and cortisol. Prolonged or excessive production of cortisol may impair cortisol binding to glucocorticoid receptors and prevent it from controlling the release of corticotropin releasing hormone (CRH). The resultant excess CRH may cause inflammation and subsequent pain. Inflammation typically results in pain because blood vessels become damaged, allowing excess water to filter from the bloodstream to the tissue so that the tissue swells and expands. The edematous tissue starts pressing against nerve endings and this pressure sends pain signals to the brain, causing discomfort (Ji *et al.* 2013).

In addition, when cortisol concentration is high over a long period of time, the adrenal glands become depleted of cortisol, leading to hypocortisolism. Hypocortisolism has been associated with low back pain and musculoskeletal pain (McEwen and Kalia 2010). A review by Hannibal and Bishop (2014) states that based on experimental evidence, it is reasonable to conclude that cortisol dysfunction, whether mediated by impaired binding to glucocorticoid receptors or adrenal depletion of cortisol, is likely to contribute to the development of chronic pain.

Muscle tension also results from stress or anxiety because when we feel stressed or anxious, our muscles naturally contract. This contraction is advantageous if you are in acute danger, but otherwise not, because tension contributes to pain and discomfort. Muscle tension is usually experienced as a dull ache, but the tension can also cause sharp and shooting pains. The pain can add to the anxiety, which in turn adds to the pain, creating a vicious circle. Tensing of muscles can lead to pain and stiffness in almost any area of the body.

Gut discomfort

Following trauma, changes often occur in the visceral organs, especially the gut. Visceral sensory nerve fibers transmit sensory information (including heat, chemical, mechanical, pain response) from the gut to the nucleus tractus solitarius in the brain stem. In addition, spinal visceral nerves transmit information about mechanical stimuli (pain) to cell bodies in the dorsal root ganglia and central terminals in the superficial dorsal horn of the spinal cord. Trauma also activates the hypothalamus-pituitary-adrenal (HPA) axis so that the hypothalamus releases CRH, which binds to receptors on the pituitary gland. This stimulates the release of adrenocorticotropic hormone, which then binds to receptors on the adrenal gland, causing release of the stress hormone, cortisol.

Chronically high concentrations of cortisol in the blood can impair many of the body's systems, especially the digestive system. As described in Chapter 6, the stress response temporarily shuts down the digestive system to conserve energy. As a result, intestinal motility is reduced, leading to constipation. Trauma can also stimulate an inflammatory response by activating immunological cells in the gut to release cytokines that damage the linings of the intestinal mucosa and associated blood vessels, leading to passage of excess water from the blood circulation into the intestinal lumen which causes diarrhea. Emotional and psychological trauma can contribute to irritable bowel syndrome, a disorder that causes abdominal pain, constipation and diarrhea (Halland et al. 2014). A model for this process is shown in Figure 7.5.

Studies by Söderholm and Perdue suggest activation of mucosal nerves, possibly releasing CRH and/or ACh, to activate mast cells (CRH may be derived from nerves or immune/inflammatory cells.) Mast cells (and possibly neurons) release bioactive chemicals (as yet not completely identified) that enhance epithelial permeability of both the transcellular and paracellular pathways.

The effect of stress on the intestinal mucosal epithelium, or lining of the gut, can be seen in Figure 7.6. The tissues were taken from rats that were either in a quiet room (Figure 7.6A) or were subjected daily to 90 dB white noise for 15 minutes (Figure 7.6B), which caused them stress (Baldwin et al. 2006). These photographs were taken by the author using electron microscopy.

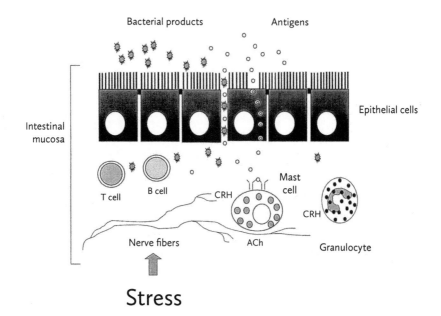

Stress

FIGURE 7.5 STRESS AND INFLAMMATION OF THE INTESTINE. SCHEMA OF
MECHANISMS INVOLVED IN STRESS-INDUCED BARRIER DYSFUNCTION.
Source: Söderholm and Perdue 2001.

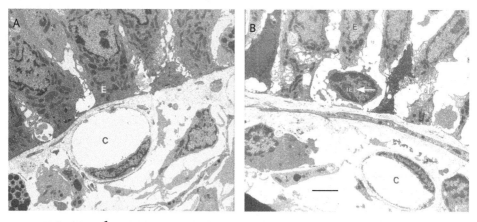

FIGURE 7.6 ELECTRON MICROGRAPHS OF MUCOSAL EPITHELIUM.
(A) In rats in the quiet room, the epithelial cells (E) generally were attached to
each other and to the basement membrane, forming a barrier. (B) In rats in the
noise room, large numbers of epithelial cells were separating from each other
and from the basement membrane, breaching the barrier. Mucosal capillaries
(C) also are visible. IEL, intraepithelial lymphocyte. Scale: 5 microns.

Although an inflammatory response is appropriate if it is triggered by harmful
bacteria or food substances in the gut, it is inappropriate if produced by emotional stress. The damage caused by the inflammatory response does not alleviate

stress in any way. In addition, stress can reduce the number of beneficial bacteria in the microbiome. Gut bacteria produce microbial metabolites that interact with intestinal enteroendocrine cells to modulate hormone secretion and expression. These hormones play key roles in regulating metabolic processes such as insulin sensitivity, glucose tolerance, fat storage and appetite. It is not surprising that the physical effects of pent-up trauma are often felt in the gut.

Information about the mechanical and chemical changes produced by stress-induced cellular responses is transmitted to the insula via the viscero-sensory pathways, which then alerts the amygdala. People who suffer from PTSD often have an overactive amygdala combined with an underactive prefrontal cortex (Badura-Brack *et al.* 2018). This makes it understandable why someone with PTSD might feel anxious around something even slightly related to the original trauma that led to the PTSD. For these patients, it is time to rebalance the ANS by stimulating the vagus nerve.

SOMATIC THERAPY

In somatic therapy, physical stimuli such as touch, movement and controlled breathing are used to stimulate the vagal complex, promote relaxation and encourage release of the physical and emotional tension associated with the trauma. The client is asked to think about the traumatic events that led to the high levels of emotional stress and then is taught to diminish the arousal through body awareness techniques and conversation. The practitioner helps clients develop resources within themselves to regulate their emotions and shift from the fight/flight/freeze response to a higher-functioning mode where they can think more clearly. The goal is to help release the client from whatever is preventing them from fully engaging in their lives.

Somatic therapy can help clients who suffer from a wide range of issues, including stress, anxiety, chronic pain, depression, grief, addiction and sexual dysfunction. Somatic therapy can be integrated into physical therapy, psychotherapy and counselling practices. There is no official accreditation for somatic therapy and so it is most important to look for someone with experience in the practice and with whom you feel comfortable discussing personal issues. However, some practitioners have Somatic Experiencing (SE™) professional training, a continuing education program developed by Peter Levine, PhD, that provides a theoretical framework for understanding and addressing trauma physiology and teaches practical skills that can be integrated into their professional practice.

Somatic therapy techniques

Here are some of the more common techniques used by somatic therapists to help release the effects of trauma from the body.

Body awareness

This is one of the first steps in learning to release tension from the body. The client learns to recognize and identify areas of tension in the body, as well as calming thoughts and feelings. The vagus nerve is the main pathway for conveying information about the internal condition of the body to the brain. Through body awareness, or interoception, we know when our heart is beating fast, when we need to take a deep breath, and when we are hot, cold, nauseous, tired or alert. Awareness of one's own bodily feelings and vagal activation seem to be of central importance for the effective regulation of emotional responses (Pinna and Edwards 2020).

Body scan

This is a mindfulness exercise that you can do by yourself, in a quiet space where you can sit or lie down comfortably for some time between five and 30 minutes. The instructions in Box 7.1 are from Laura K. Schenck, PhD, LPC, a licensed professional counsellor with a doctorate in counselling psychology from the University of Northern Colorado. As you read each set of instructions, pause to become more attuned to your body without judgment, simply increasing curious awareness of your physical sensations and the experience itself.

BOX 7.1 BODY SCAN

Find a comfortable position, seated or lying down, where your body feels at ease and supported by the ground, chair or cushion beneath you.

First, bring your attention to your breath. Notice the sensation of the air as you inhale through your nostrils, and again as you exhale through your mouth.

Pause to make room for whatever you may be feeling, including tension or discomfort.

Now, start at your feet by bringing your awareness to the physical sensations present in your feet, calves, knees and thighs. Notice the sensations in your muscles as you allow your mindful focus to slowly move upward.

If you notice any areas of tension or holding during this body scan, pause to mindfully attend to this tension, then deliberately allow the tension to dissipate and release.

Next, take a deep breath in as you bring awareness to sensations present in your abdomen, torso and lower back. Notice your spine as you gradually allow your focus to continually move upward along your body, remembering to pause at any areas of tension or holding, allowing those areas to gently relax.

Maintain a focus on the rhythm of your breath as you slowly breathe in... and slowly breathe out...allowing any physical discomfort to be released as you slowly exhale...imagining the tension dissolve with each out-breath.

Continue to allow your focus to continue upwards, noticing your hands, arms, elbows and shoulders. Become awareness of any tightness, discomfort or holding in these areas. Use the gentle flow of your breath to bring your awareness to these areas and allow them to release as you slowly and gently exhale.

Finally, bring your attention to your neck, face and head. Notice the sensations present in your jaw, mouth and eyes. Allow any areas of tension to relax, noticing the tension melt away as you bring your mindful awareness to these areas.

Grounding

This is the act of connecting deeply to your body and the earth. Grounding involves sensing the body, feeling your feet on the ground and breathing more deeply and slowly than usual to calm your nervous system.

Orientation

As indicated by Peter Levine, orientation is the natural response of animals to scan the environment to assess it for safety. This requires agility to turn the head so that the eyes, ears and nose can orient toward the source of stimulation and either respond to it as a potential threat or remain calm if all is safe. These responses utilize the optic and oculomotor cranial branches of the vagus system. When orientation is used in somatic therapy, clients are encouraged to pay attention to the sensations in their body that may arise as they notice the objects in the room. The vagus nerve is responsible for providing somatic sensation information for the skin behind the ear, the external part of the ear canal and certain parts of the throat, supplying visceral sensation information for the larynx, esophagus, lungs, trachea, heart and most of the digestive tract.

If the client finds it difficult to access their body sensations, they may be asked to name the items that they observe around them. This simple process will engage the facial and hypoglossal cranial branches of the vagus system and will also engage the prefrontal cortex, the thinking part of the brain, and decrease stimulation of the amygdala, reducing the "fight or flight" response. In Box 7.2 is an orientation exercise you can do by yourself if you are entering a new environment. It is based on teachings by Gloria Gonzales, CMT SEP, who is founder of the Institute for Somatic Education and Integrative Wellness.

BOX 7.2 ORIENTATION EXERCISE

Out in the world, your body automatically assesses your surroundings for safety, often without your conscious awareness.

Sit or stand in this environment. Become conscious, taking special note of your feet and "back body" as you do so (back body = back of head, back of the spine, gluteal muscles (buttocks), hamstrings and back heels).

Now allow your eyes to rest and for their awareness to rest and recede back toward the center of the brain. Allow your face to soften.

Slowly now, let your eyes and senses gently scan the environment. Notice an object, color or a shape of particular interest. Let your senses rest there for a bit without locking in. Let your eyes and the whole of your body "receive" rather than "retrieve" the things within your environment. Sit back and receive the sense of your environment.

"Receive" is the key word.

Now notice internal body sensations that arise from engaging in this way. Notice the other ways in which your body responds to the present moment in a safe, secure and open way.

Now notice your body and breath. You may experience ease, quietude, softness, fullness or centeredness.

Pendulation

In this technique, a therapist guides you from a relaxed state to one that more resembles your traumatic experience. This may be repeated several times, allowing you to release the pent-up tension. As the tension is released, you may feel uncomfortable or anxious. Each time, you will be guided back to a relaxed state. Over time, you will learn to shift to a relaxed state on your own.

Titration

In this technique, the therapist guides you through a traumatic memory. You will be asked to observe any changes in your body that you sense as you describe the memory. If you experience any physical sensations, the therapist will help you address them as they occur.

Sequencing

This involves paying close attention to the order in which sensations of tension leave your body. For instance, first you might feel release of a tightening in your chest and then from your throat. There may be a sensation of trembling during the process.

Resourcing

This involves recalling resources in your life that make you feel safe, such as your relationships, including with pets; your character strengths; your home or a favorite place. It can include anything that makes you feel calm and secure.

You then relive the good feelings and sensations associated with your resources, which act as an emotional anchor.

Some additional physical techniques that may be used with somatic therapy include dance, exercise, yoga, meditation, vocal work (humming, singing, chanting) and "bodywork." Bodywork involves a therapist working with the motion of your body or face and perhaps manipulating your tissue, as with massage or physical therapy.

Physical therapy

Physical therapists are trained to evaluate musculoskeletal impairments which may contribute to pain and loss of function. Treatment interventions are usually a combination of patient education, manual therapy techniques to mobilize tissue restriction and exercises or neuromotor reeducation to restore normal strength and movement patterns. Patient somatosensory awareness is important to optimize physical therapy progress towards goals. Anecdotally, physical therapists occasionally encounter patients whose progress is impeded due to suboptimal somatosensory awareness. For example, during exercise instruction or manual stretching sessions, the physical therapist will use a specific technique to obtain a predetermined range of motion during a stretch; the therapist's goal is to teach the patient to reproduce the technique independently. However, patients will report difficulty "feeling" a specific muscle, whether it has increased tension or is able to release tension. A common therapy scenario involves a physical therapist encouraging a patient "to just relax" as the therapist tries to stretch or mobilize a restricted body part; the patient will say "I am" in frustration. Both the therapist and the patient become frustrated; patients may discontinue therapy sessions, and the therapist may incorrectly label the patient as "non-compliant."

Nervous system dysregulation is often seen as having difficulty "staying present" during physical therapy sessions or having difficulty following exercise programs/lifestyle modifications as prescribed by the physical therapist. Patients are observed being in a sympathetic nervous system state (fight or flight). In a sympathetic nervous system state, muscle tone is often increased and patients "have difficulty feeling muscular tension" while providers are doing manual therapy techniques. Patients also may hold their breath while trying to perform stretches or exercises. Physical therapy patient education ideally would include somatosensory awareness techniques to increase the patient's ability to increase vagus nerve activation and therefore increase parasympathetic activity.

The vagus nerve includes two parts: the dorsal vagal complex (DVC), or dorsal motor nucleus (freeze response), and ventral vagal complex (calm activation).

Dr. Stephen Porges, who developed the polyvagal theory, found that the ventral vagus nerve operated as a third state between sympathetic activation and the dorsal freeze response: the social engagement system, or a social nervous system. He also found that there was a defense system hierarchy. A person is unconsciously moving through stages of autonomic activation throughout the day. Where one is in the stages of activation depends on whether one feels safe or one's safety feels threatened.

CASE STUDY: Mind-body integration for improved sexual function
Diana Fassett, PT, SEP, Physical Therapist, Somatic Experiencing Practitioner, Success Physical Therapy, Tucson, AZ (successphysicaltherapy.com)

Introduction
The following case study describes a course of physical therapy working on self-regulation of the autonomic nervous system; specifically, increasing patient somatic awareness of sympathetic activation and techniques to return to a parasympathetic state. The treatment sessions focused on supporting the patient's use of orientation to his extrinsic and intrinsic environment to allow a pendulation shift from sympathetic activation and return to parasympathetic state.

The patient "JL" is a 61-year-old married male with self-diagnosed erectile dysfunction; he seeks treatment from a pelvic floor physical therapist with training as a Somatic Experiencing practitioner. Somatic Experiencing sessions invite the patient/client in contemplation of an experience as having sensation, meaning, images, emotions, and at times behaviors. Contemplation of these components, especially the somatic or body sensation awareness while learning skills to "stay present," often helps clients to renegotiate trauma experiences.

Treatment sessions took place in a physical therapy treatment room, seated across from JL in comfortable chairs of choice. The room was decorated with various items of potential interest to offer options for curiosity and orientation. JL was encouraged to position his chair at a distance that met his sense of a comfortable distance from mine.

Initial session
The initial session is history taking. JL describes a loving supportive relationship with his spouse who has previously experienced pelvic pain and dyspareunia (pain with penetration), now since resolved with pelvic floor physical therapy.

As JL contemplates return to penetrative intercourse with his spouse, he has experienced "performance anxiety" and suboptimal penile tumescence (erection) to allow penetration. Patient education includes psycho-education regarding autonomic nervous system, sympathetic and parasympathetic nervous system branches, and the ability of the body to move back and forth between the two states.

Education is provided regarding my role in sessions; to offer gentle interruption of sympathetic response prior to escalation beyond threshold (to prevent JL from moving into a dorsal ventral state overwhelm or "freeze"). More specific patient education is also provided regarding pelvic floor muscle function and the sexual arousal process. Sexual arousal has been determined to be a parasympathetic response. "Anxiety" and fear/anticipation of failure may cause a sympathetic response during sexual activity, resulting in lack of adequate erectile response (tumescence).

The key to creating an erectile response is the dominance of parasympathetic activity that results in cavernosal artery (also known as the deep artery of the penis) smooth muscle relaxation allowing erection to occur, over the tonic, sympathetically driven smooth muscle and blood vessel contraction responsible for flaccidity (Prieto 2008).

The initial evaluation session was notable for JL expressing "nervousness" as we discussed his sense of the unknown regarding physical therapy intervention. We also discussed his frustration and conflict between how much he loves his wife and, at the same time, not understanding why his body is not responding adequately.

JL was encouraged to notice his current somatosensory experience; he was able to identify muscular tension and increased breathing rate (sympathetic response) as he reflected on his stressful experiences or "unpleasant" feelings. JL was then invited to use orientation skills to "notice" items of interest in the room; he could relate a pleasant story or emotion to these items at times. I would then invite him to pause and "notice" where in his body he might feel any particular sensations or body experience. Of particular interest or curiosity would be his awareness of "shifts or changes" in the perceived level of intensity of the body sensations. I explained to JL that each person's somatic experience is different; for example, sadness may present as a "heaviness," whereas a more positive emotion may be described as "lightness" or "openness." We discussed unpleasant emotions such as guilt, shame, embarrassment and anger; JL was able to notice the physical somatic sensations also seemed unpleasant. In comparison, his pleasant emotions such as happy, energized or excited seemed to be noticed as pleasant somatic sensations in his body.

Typically, patients will initially notice items of interest that are more pleasant, and when encouraged to identify the detail regarding the pleasant observation, patients are then invited to notice if there is an area of the body that may seem to have shifted in its tension level (from sympathetic response to a more parasympathetic state). The goal is to practice moving in gentle pendulation between sympathetic and parasympathetic states while supporting the patient to prevent moving into a dorsal vagal state.

I was able to support several cycles of pendulation with JL during the first session; JL then commented his "legs felt more settled and less restless." Breathing rate also returned to baseline; he actually yawned. JL was given homework of visualization and gratitude observations on a daily basis; goals were to notice physical tensions in his body or emotions as they might arise. He was already an active meditator and was encouraged to notice his somatosensory response at both the beginning and at the end of meditation sessions.

Additional sessions
JL was seen for four additional sessions, once every two weeks for eight weeks. Sessions would begin with orientation to the therapy room; JL initially would tend to drift quickly into sympathetic response. Education and contemplation of the tendency to drift towards negative vs positive thought processes were utilized, and JL was encouraged to notice without judgment. Multiple vagus nerve stimulation techniques were used during the sessions, including humming or vocalizing to create vibration in the vocal cords during exhale.

JL was able to notice a shift in somatosensory awareness, from tension during sympathetic activation, to a sense of relaxation or "relief" as tension resolved. JL was able to generalize and discuss his awareness of this experience during sexual encounters at home; he was able to progress to noticing his negative thought process of anticipation of failure; and through his practice of checking in and "noticing" his body sensations, he was able to allow return to parasympathetic instead of letting negative emotion take over and continue to body tension, which used to result in sympathetic response and suboptimal or inability to achieve erectile response.

Last session
At his last session, JL reported he and his wife were "back to normal." He expressed gratitude for support of his therapy process and was looking forward

to continuing his plan of care independently. Of note, JL contacted me over a year later requesting to come in for a "tune up"; he said he was having some trouble again and wanted to do a session. An appointment was set, but JL then contacted me a few days later and said he had been able to talk to his wife and review some stresses that had come up; he realized the stresses were affecting his ability to use his therapy tools. He was able to review and "get himself back on his previous plan of care with success."

In summary, somatic awareness skills helped JL learn to stay aware of his extrinsic stresses and intrinsic body responses. He was able to notice when the body responses were beginning; he was able to utilize his tools (humming, orienting, breathing, stretches and meditation/visualization) to stimulate his vagus nerve for parasympathetic response and prevent compromise/impairments to his sexual function.

REFERENCES

Badura-Brack A, McDermott TJ, Heinrichs-Graham E et al., 2018. Veterans with PTSD demonstrate amygdala hyperactivity while viewing threatening faces: a MEG study. *Biol Psychol.* 132: 228–232. doi: 10.1016/j.biopsycho.2018.01.005.

Baldwin AL, Primeau RL and Johnson WE, 2006. Effect of noise on the morphology of the intestinal mucosa in laboratory rats. *J Am Assoc Lab Anim Sci.* 45(1): 74-82.

Halland M, Almazar A, Lee R et al., 2014. A case-control study of childhood and adult trauma in the development of irritable bowel syndrome (IBS). *Neurogastroenterol Motil.* 26(7): 990–998. doi: 10.1111/nmo.12353.

Hannibal KE and Bishop MD, 2014. Chronic stress, cortisol dysfunction, and pain: a psychoneuroendocrine rationale for stress management in pain rehabilitation. *Phys Ther.* 94(12): 1816–1825. doi: 10.2522/ptj.20130597.

Ji G, Fu Y, Adwanikar H and Neugebauer V, 2013. Non-pain-related CRF1 activation in the amygdala facilitates synaptic transmission and pain responses. *Mol Pain.* 9: 2. doi: 10.1186/1744-8069-9-2.

Kabat-Zinn J, 2003. Mindfulness-based interventions in context: past, present, and future. *Clinical Psychology: Science and Practice.* 10(2): 144–156. doi: 10.1093/clipsy.bpg016.

Lagattuta KH, Elrod NM and Kramer HJ, 2016. How do thoughts, emotions, and decisions align? A new way to examine theory of mind during middle childhood and beyond. *J Exp Child Psychol.* 149: 116–133. doi: 10.1016/j.jecp.2016.01.013.

McEwen BS and Kalia M, 2010. The role of corticosteroids and stress in chronic pain conditions. *Metabolism.* 59(suppl 1): S9–S15. doi: 10.1016/j.metabol.2010.07.012.

Pinna T and Edwards DJ, 2020. A systematic review of associations between interoception, vagal tone, and emotional regulation: potential applications for mental health, wellbeing, psychological flexibility, and chronic conditions. *Front Psychol.* 11: 1792. doi: 10.3389/fpsyg.2020.01792.

Prieto D, 2008. Physiological regulation of penile arteries and veins. *Int J Impot Res.* 20(1): 17– 29. doi: 10.1038/sj.ijir.3901581.

Söderholm JD and Perdue MH, 2001. Stress and gastrointestinal tract. II. Stress and intestinal barrier function. *Am J Physiol Gastrointest Liver Physiol.* 280(1): G7–G13. doi: 10.1152/ajpgi.2001.280.1.G7.

CHAPTER 8

Powering Up Your Vagus Nerve

HOW HORSES PROVIDE BIOFEEDBACK

INTRODUCTION

In this book so far, we have explored various ways of activating the vagus nerve and which types of therapists can support and guide you for each method in this endeavor. In this chapter, we go one step further and consider not only how vagal stimulation benefits *you* but also how it enhances your relationships with others. Although horses are not humans, Equine Assisted Learning (EAL) provides a unique opportunity to practice techniques such as the body scan, heart-focused coherent breathing and sensual awareness in the presence of another living being, and discover how you can influence their willingness to engage with you in a non-judgmental way.

For this work to be effective, there is no need for participants to ride the horses. All the benefits of horse–human connection can be achieved while participants are standing on the ground. Experienced horse men and women know that the way they breathe affects their horse's behavior. Horses, as non-predatory animals, are continually aware of their environment, and as you watch them, they provide instant feedback to you based on your behavior, your body language and the emotions you are feeling and emanating. A horse usually responds more favorably to a person who breathes slowly and deeply, compared to one who, perhaps out of fear or anxiety, shows up with fast, shallow breathing. By observing how the horses respond to you and by noticing your own bodily sensations and emotions in the present moment, you can learn how to regulate your ANS using vagal stimulation skills. Our research has shown that when people are in a balanced autonomic state, which we call "coherence" or "relaxed alertness," horses are much more likely to engage and interact with them.

In this chapter, we will start with a little history of the horse–human connection and then move on to the importance of working with an experienced and qualified EAL facilitator, or guide. Some direction will be given regarding the various types of programs that are available and the certifications that designate a practitioner's proficiency. Next, we will describe how you can use your breath as a language to alter a horse's behavior, illustrated by an example from an experienced horse trainer and by results from scientific research. Just imagine, if you can successfully use your breath to influence the behavior of a 1500-pound animal, what can you do with another person?

Social engagement is another technique to activate the vagal system. We will demonstrate, using a case study, that horses can facilitate social engagement, both between horses and humans and between humans. Finally, we will discuss neuroception, a concept based on the polyvagal theory, which posits that neural circuits can distinguish whether situations or people may be safe, dangerous or life-threatening and then attune your physiology and behavior to cope with these situations. How does this apply to horses? Through their evolution, horses have become very skilled at evaluating situations regarding safety and danger, and at responding appropriately. We will demonstrate, using a case study, that a person who has experienced trauma in the past can become more proficient at regulating their own ANS and at responding to situations in a more appropriate manner, by observing how a horse responds to them when they activate their ventral vagus complex and signal "safety" to the horse.

A LITTLE HISTORY

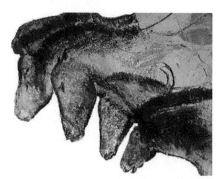

FIGURE 8.1 HORSE PAINTING
ON THE WALLS OF CHAUVET
CAVE, ARDÈCHE, FRANCE.
*Source: Wolfgang Ruppert/
Art Resource, New York.*

Thirty-two thousand years ago some unknown people drew a collection of remarkable pictures of animals, many of them horses, on the walls of the Chauvet Cave in France (Figure 8.1). One particularly striking picture is a painting of a group of four horses. Rather than looking like a herd, the picture seems to represent a detailed study of horses in different attitudes; one horse has his lips parted as if neighing. It appears that these artists from an earlier era were concerned with closely observing the horses and wanted to make sure that their artwork accurately reflected the spirit and behavior of horses.

THE IMPORTANCE OF A GUIDE

Horses are large animals that can have it in their nature to be unpredictable, so it is essential that EAL is performed under the guidance of an equine professional and an EAL facilitator. Professional Association of Therapeutic Horsemanship standards and guidelines should be followed in all situations. In this way, EAL provides a safe and secure opportunity for real-life practice of self-regulation skills as well as the possibility of forming social bonds with the horses and other participants. In addition, the presence of an experienced equine professional to guide the horse–human interaction is especially important because the development of an attachment bond between horse and human depends on the behavior of the participant, not just of the horse.

Even experienced horse-owners do not always reach a state of ventral vagal activation after interacting with their horse. We know this because a colleague of mine, Barbara K. Rector MA, LLC, Certified Equine International Professional, ran a pilot study at a semi-private training and teaching ranch where she boarded her horse. Sixteen fellow boarders, all adults, consented to the study in which Barbara measured their HRV before and after they engaged with their horse in ordinary equine-related activities such as grooming and riding. Most people rode rather than groomed. After interacting with their horses, only six participants showed an overall increase in HRV (measured as SDNN). A boost in SDNN in a healthy person after engaging in an activity usually indicates a more balanced autonomic state. Only eight participants showed an increase in the parasympathetic, or vagal component of HRV (measured as RMSSD). As described in Chapter 2, RMSSD reflects the parasympathetic component of HRV because it only includes very fast beat-to-beat changes in HRV, instead of the more gradual changes that take several heartbeats or longer to establish themselves.

Comments collected from the participants in answer to a questionnaire indicated that their experience was not always positive regarding their emotional responses. For example, a few participants were worried about their horse's health or subpar performance, and this was worsened by the interaction. Another was anxious about an upcoming show. In these cases, an equine professional or EAL facilitator would have noticed these feelings and given the participant the opportunity to express and release them using vagal stimulating techniques, such as body scans or changes in breathing, reinforced by feedback from the horse. Left to our own devices, this important step is often ignored or forgotten.

Equine Assisted Learning programs and certification

A professional certification is a credential that verifies someone's knowledge, skill and abilities to perform a specific job. Certifications are usually awarded by a professional association after a candidate completes an assessment of some kind.

Professional Association of Therapeutic Horsemanship, PATH International "certifies and accredits centers, instructors and equine specialists according to a set of field-tested standards to ensure the highest levels of safety, ethics and effectiveness in the equine-assisted services industry. Instructors must complete workshops and pass both written and practical exams to become certified to teach equine-assisted services. Participants and their families can be confident that PATH International Member Centers and Professionals deliver safe and effective equine assisted services programming."

A PATH International Equine Specialist in Mental Health and Learning (ESMHL) "ensures the safety and well-being of the equine participating in equine-facilitated mental health and learning sessions. The ESMHL serves as the equine expert during equine/human interactions and works with mental health or education providers to ethically incorporate equines in their practice, within the scope of their profession. An ESMHL must be knowledgeable in horsemanship and understands how to collaborate with a mental health therapist and/or educator to best meet the client's needs and keep the lesson safe."

Equine Assisted Growth and Learning Association (EAGALA) "certifies both mental health professionals as well as horse specialists through its certification program. To become certified, a person must complete an online course, attend an onsite training program, pass an exam, and submit a professional portfolio."

The HERD Institute° offers "Equine-Facilitated Psychotherapy & Learning Certifications for mental health practitioners, coaches, educators, and training professionals." Their training focuses on teaching students the philosophical, theoretical and experiential process of incorporating equines into work with their specific client populations. Their certification programs are offered through a hybrid of online and in-person training available throughout the USA, Canada, and the UK.

EAQ° **– Home of Horse-based Learning and Education** "sets and monitors quality standards for its equine assisted learning centers and provides training and qualifications for facilitators and others involved with equine assisted learning. There is a number of EAQ Approved Centers in the UK offering interaction with horses for children, young people and adults leading to nationally recognized qualifications." EAQ offers training programs for facilitators including the Level 4 Certificate in Facilitating Equine Assisted Learning which is a national qualification that is regulated in the UK by the Office of Qualifications and Examinations Regulation, Ofqual.

BREATHING AS A LANGUAGE

Advice from a horse trainer

Everyone has heard the term "horse whisperer," but horse whisperers are not actually whispering; they are regulating their breath as they interact with the horse. Their breathing is a way of having a conversation with the horse. One person is so convinced of this phenomenon that he teaches it to medical students. He is Allan J. Hamilton, MD (Figure 8.2). Dr Hamilton, a personal colleague of mine, is a Harvard-trained brain surgeon, professor of neurosurgery at the University of Arizona, a renowned horse trainer, developer of EAL programs and the author of *Zen Mind, Zen Horse*.

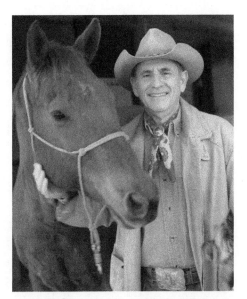

FIGURE 8.2 ALLAN J. HAMILTON, MD.
Source: Courtesy of Allan J. Hamilton.
www.storey.com/books/lead-with-your-heart-lessons-from-a-life-with-horses.

BOX 8.1 ADVICE FROM A HORSE TRAINER

As a horse trainer, the greatest tool I have for communicating directly with any horse is my breathing. To create clarity of mind, I use my breathing because it is the key to creating an active versus a passive energy state. Applying active energy to my horse makes him respond with physical action. Shifting to passive energy slows him down, rewards him, or brings him to a stop.

Why is breath so central? Because the horse is trying to sense what our body language and posture are telling him, the amount of energy stored in our body as tension is an important cue to him.

Take a breath right now. Gulp it in on purpose. Now hold your breath for a moment. Feel how it suddenly brings tension into your frame, almost making you rigid? That's what your horse can feel when you hold your breath. And after training horse owners and trainers, ninety percent or more, hold their breath and take shorter gulps when they work with their horse. Okay, now let the air out. You can feel your whole musculoskeletal frame sag and let go. That's an energetic release inside your own body. Energetic release is what tells a horse to relax. It's a reward. So, breathe in: my body tenses to indicate I am asking my horse to do something: to move, jump, pick up a lead, accelerate his gait. Breathe out. Relax. It's over. You've done what I asked. Slow down. Stop moving your feet and come stand by me. Every transition up or down is accompanied by a change in my breath. In between transitions, I try to breathe regularly. I use my breath control for any change up or down in the energy I am applying to my horse.

How do you practice breath control? Start with something simple like grooming your horse. Use your breath as you're brushing him. Use your breathing – long deep expirations – to help him to relax his frame. Once you're ready to lead him off, breathe in, energy up, get him moving out with you. Get to the gate, breathe out because you want him to stop at the gate. Just start linking in your own brain that you need to be mindful when you are increasing or decreasing the amount of energy or pressure you are positing on the horse.

Finally, take that breath control and extend the lesson to your life. When you're getting ready to do a presentation, breathe out and relax. Before you start, energize. Breathe in. Listening to your teenage kids? Tempted to interrupt? Be judgmental? Breathe out. Relax your body to make your mind clear so you are listening attentively. Working with horses is one of the easiest ways I know how to teach people to become mindful of their breath because horses are so exquisitely sensitive to the energy we transmit in our bodies.

Source: Courtesy of Hamilton AJ, 2016. How every breath you take is affecting your horse and his training. www.horsetalk. co.nz/2016/09/26/breath-affecting-horse-training.

SCIENTIFIC RESEARCH STUDIES

I have worked for the last 12 years with a small group of colleagues on a multiphase project to explore the horse–human connection. Our objective is to monitor physiological changes experienced by horses and humans as they engage with each other during specific EAL exercises. We are searching for answers to the following questions:

- Are these physiological changes mutually beneficial?
- Is there any synchronicity in these changes between the horse and the human?
- Are horse and human exchanging physiological information?

Details of some of the research studies have been published (Baldwin *et al.* 2018, 2021, 2023). A summary of some of the overall results is given in the following section, focusing mainly on the effects of breath regulation on physiological and behavioral responses.

Rock back and sigh: using breath to stimulate one's ventral vagal complex when with a horse

© 2019 ANN LINDA BALDWIN, PHD, AND LINDA KOHANOV

Our original three-part study involved three groups of 24 people, age 55 or older with no horse experience. In the first two studies, we measured various physiological effects in humans while they groomed or slowly approached horses who were restrained (Baldwin *et al.* 2018) as seen in Figure 8.3.

We hypothesized that these activities, called Mindful Grooming and With Your Permission, would be relaxing. We were therefore surprised to find that heart rate increased. We also sampled saliva for immunoglobulin A (IgA) which is a protective antibody for the intestine and respiratory systems (IgA is known to decrease when the body is stressed). In these activities, IgA remained constant. This meant the activity was invigorating but not stressful. It turns out that grooming a horse wakes you up; it stimulates you in a positive way.

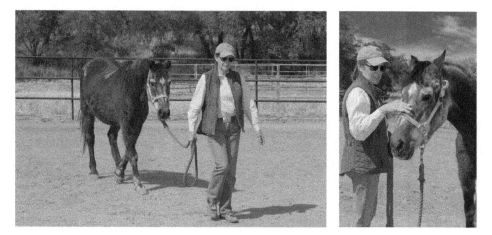

FIGURE 8.3 HORSE–HUMAN INTERACTION.

We also found that this simple activity increases your heart health. We measured heart rate variability (HRV) which is a measure of adaptability and improved cardiac function. High HRV is associated with reduced anxiety, improved memory and enhanced cognitive skills. We found that HRV not only significantly increased but shifted to the very low frequency range. A number of studies has shown that people who are deficient in the very low frequency range (0.003–0.04 Hz) of heart rate variability show increased chance of death after a heart attack (Ryan *et al.* 2011), inflammation (Lampert *et al.* 2008; Stein *et al.* 2008), post-stroke infection (Brämer *et al.* 2019) and post-traumatic stress disorder (Shah *et al.* 2013). An increase in the very low frequency range of HRV in humans would be very beneficial.

It is significant that full-sized horses have the majority of their HRV in the very low frequency range, while humans are normally in the low and high frequency ranges, with a smaller percentage in the very low frequency range. This increase of the very low frequency range in the presence of the horses was physiological evidence that people were being positively affected by these animals. We did not observe these responses in control groups who groomed a toy horse or who slowly approached humans rather than horses. Another study (unpublished) showed that people interacting with miniature horses, who are often brought into nursing homes and used as therapy horses, did not increase the very low frequency range in humans. (The miniature horses themselves did not have much HRV in the very low frequency range. They were more like humans.) We deduced from this that there are distinct health-enhancing advantages to working with full-sized horses.

In these two activities, the participants were not required to alter the horse's behavior in any way because the horse was either tied for grooming or held on a lead rope by an experienced horse handler. In therapeutic and leadership contexts, these studies showed that simply grooming or mindfully approaching a gentle restrained horse has significant benefits for stress reduction, heart health and clear thinking. We often encounter clients from all walks of life who are ambitious, "type A" personalities, and highly stressed. A simple task like grooming is a good place to start.

As a next step, we wanted to study activities designed to alter the horse's behavior. Social intelligence and leadership skills involve connecting and influencing others as well as building trust and breaking through resistance. So, with the next activity, we upped the ante in several ways. This time, the horse was loose, milling around at liberty in a sizable corral. The goal was to attract the horse's attention, have the horse come to you and voluntarily walk with you (Figure 8.4).

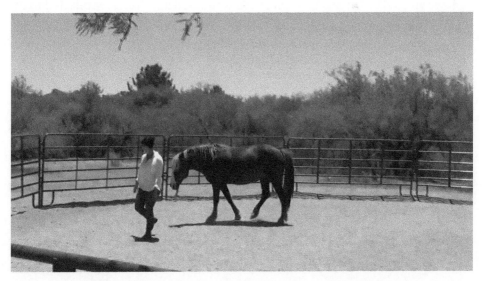

FIGURE 8.4 A HORSE VOLUNTARILY WALKING WITH A CLIENT.

As a result of the previous two studies, we hypothesized that the activity would also increase heart rate, overall heart rate variability and the very low frequency

HRV component. This third activity, Leadership through Connection, involved mindfully approaching a loose horse and noticing when the horse showed body language that he was alert to the human's presence. This usually consists of ear movements and posture shifts resulting from a mild increase in stress as the horse's autonomic nervous system notices there's something new in the environment – in this case, a human walking over to him. We call this a "proximity response."

The human is then taught to rock back slightly and sigh, which is a long, relaxed outbreath. We had previously noticed that unrestrained horses will walk away from people who are holding their breath and are attracted to people as they audibly exhale. At first, we didn't know why this occurred from a physiological perspective. We also didn't know why some horses merely looked curiously at a person in response to the exhale, while others walked toward the individual, and even followed them. The study results gave us some very interesting answers to these questions.

As expected, during and after this activity, the heart rate of participants increased, but the IgA remained constant. This meant the activity was invigorating but not stressful. Unlike in the previous two studies, however, neither HRV nor the very low frequency component significantly changed. At first, we were surprised by these results. We then wondered if it may be connected to the extra challenge of working with a loose horse.

To gain some insight, we went back to a previous pilot test in which one of our research partners, Linda Kohanov, had her HRV recorded while interacting with a loose horse. The HRV monitor was synchronized with a video camera so that we could see if the HRV was correlated with the horse's behavior. We noticed that the horse would look at Linda when she rocked back and sighed but would only approach her when her HRV showed a specific wavelike pattern, which was not evident at other times. This wavelike pattern represents a state of *coherence* in which the sympathetic and parasympathetic components are in perfect harmony.

In the previous studies with grooming or mindfully approaching a horse, the HRV increased but did not show the wavelike coherent pattern. Coherence is a more balanced, highly productive state. When people are coherent, they can take in more information and perform at a higher level. Memory and cognitive function improve, as does problem-solving ability. The heart and the immune system work more efficiently. Anxiety, stress and emotions are much better regulated. Benefits also include increased access to intuition and creativity, and favorable changes in hormonal balance. The person is in a state of "relaxed alertness" and is ready for anything. It's like playing tennis and waiting for the serve. You're right in front of the net on the center of the court, prepared to move in any direction. You are "in the zone."

Once we realized the possible importance of coherence, we performed multiple pilot tests with different horses and people, many of whom had little or no horse experience, in which the HRV monitor was synchronized with a video camera. We specifically taught the humans how to become coherent so we could see how it affected the horse's behavior. Repeatedly, horses would walk over to a person when he or she became coherent.

Linda "accidentally" learned how to cultivate coherence through interacting with lots of different horses and being rewarded for accessing this state unconsciously through positive feedback from each horse. Analyzing the video, she realized that when she became coherent, she was moving more fluidly in what she called "a relaxed yet heightened awareness" while breathing more deeply and evenly. She described a state of "interpersonal mindfulness," paying attention to her own non-verbal communication and its effect on the horse, making subtle adjustments from moment to moment, while sending the horse positive, inviting feelings. From this experience, we suspect that "horse whisperers" and other gifted animal trainers are unknowingly achieving this state in a similar way.

As it turns out, it is not difficult to teach people how to become coherent. The Institute of HeartMath has developed the Quick Coherence® Technique which can be practiced in order to reach the coherent state (Box 8.2).

BOX 8.2 QUICK COHERENCE® TECHNIQUE

Step 1: Focus your attention in the area of the heart. Imagine your breath is flowing in and out of your heart or chest area, breathing a little more slowly and deeply than usual.

Step 2: Make a sincere attempt to experience a regenerative feeling, such as appreciation or care for someone or something in your life.

Source: Quick Coherence® is a registered trademark of Quantum Intech, Inc. (dba HeartMath Inc.). For all HeartMath Trademarks go to www.heartmath.com/trademarks.

Based on these previous studies and pilot tests, we decided to investigate the role of coherence in leadership through a two-session pilot program. We chose six people who were more experienced with horses and familiar with the Leadership through Connection activity so that we could remove the variables of performance anxiety and the apprehension novices encounter during their early experiences with a loose horse. Most of these participants were over 55 years old, but all were over 30. Although none had been taught to access the coherent state, all had leadership experience, often in an entrepreneurial context. Once again, their heart rate variability was monitored as they performed the activity, and the whole process was video recorded.

Similar to all the previous studies, heart rate significantly increased during the process. The HRV *did* increase while performing the activity, but not statistically significantly. However, the initial resting heart rate variability of these participants was 33 percent higher than the novices. We are not sure why this is, but this group had spent much more time with horses and had gone through an in-depth equine-facilitated leadership program.

During part one of the pilot, there was a trend toward a shift to the very low frequency component of HRV. Finally, even though they had just been taught how to become coherent on the day of the study, all showed the wavelike HRV pattern intermittently during their interactions, and these instances coincided with the horse showing interest, walking toward the human and sometimes "following the leader."

Everyone commented that it was challenging at first to access coherence while performing an activity that involved paying attention to the non-verbal cues of others. To reliably attract the horse to engage and follow, people had to maintain a state of inner focus and outer focus simultaneously. The best results on video were achieved when the human was able to be coherent while at the same time pay full attention to the horse.

This same group was tested again six months later. During that time, they had practiced adding coherence to the Leadership through Connection protocol. The changes were impressive:

- They came in with a 17 percent higher *resting* HRV. This means their status quo heart health, mental clarity and emotional stability had improved, positively impacting all aspects of their lives.
- During the activity they maintained this high heart rate variability. This time, however, the percentage of HRV in the very low frequency range *doubled* during the activity. The change was highly statistically significant.

These results indicate that the horse was having a huge influence on the human's nervous system, suggesting a deeper, more profound connection between the two. The health benefits of shifting the human's HRV to the very low frequency range would include decreased chance of death after a heart attack, reduced chronic inflammation and a reduced chance of developing PTSD after a traumatic event.

Breathing as a language

During this last phase of the study, we realized that people were engaging various tools naturally, according to the needs of the situation and the horse. These include the rock back and sigh, coherent breathing and another predictably effective technique we called "the surge." The latter is a long outbreath combined with an energetic, sweeping movement that draws the horse forward, as a canoe naturally falls into the wake of a motorboat.

Neither the rock back and sigh nor the surge was coherent, but they were useful in different instances to motivate the horse to connect and follow. All three had different HRV signatures. The long outbreath associated with rock back and sigh helped a nervous or distracted horse to relax and connect. The surge helped to energize a horse who was stuck or starting to lose momentum. Combining all three as needed created a non-verbal language that enhanced communication between horse and human, creating a flowing dance of connection, rather than a pattern of jerky stops and starts.

Over time, people practicing these skills learned to consciously process and respond to (rather than unconsciously react to) non-verbal information coming from themselves and others. In effect, they were processing silent cues from the horse, then altering their own physiology to influence the horse's behavior. This skill was easily translated to human situations – for example, engaging people who were frightened, aggressive or shut down more easily, or helping to change the tone of a group in a more productive direction.

Insight into polyvagal theory helped us to understand how these three tools work together. The polyvagal theory is based on three evolutionary stages of the autonomic nervous system, the part of the nervous system that maintains organ function. The first is a primitive "dorsal vagus" nerve that fosters digestion and responds to threat by depressing metabolic activity. The second is a "sympathetic" nervous system that increases metabolic output and inhibits the dorsal vagus to engage behaviors necessary for "fight or flight." The third, and most recent is a "ventral vagus" nerve that *can rapidly regulate cardiac output* to foster engagement and disengagement with the environment. The vagus nerve is anatomically linked to nerves that regulate social engagement through facial expression and vocalization, the "ventral vagal complex."

From a polyvagal informed perspective, the rock back and sigh stimulates the ventral vagal complex in mammals, which encourages relaxation and social connection. Coherence reflects an alternating stimulation of the parasympathetic and sympathetic nerves to create a state of relaxed alertness. The surge raises energy by stimulating the sympathetic nerves, and at the same time engages connectivity by stimulating the ventral vagal complex.

Conclusion

So how can this research on horse–human interactions help you become a better leader? Well, first, being able to achieve a state of coherence puts you in a relaxed alert state that inhibits you from wasting emotional energy and sharpens your cognition. You are able to come up with novel solutions to problems that previously seemed insoluble. Not only that – you are now able to fully engage with people and show them that they matter. When you are coherent, you become more approachable because you have opened up a space in your life, in that moment, to allow for connection with another being. However, just being coherent is usually not enough to maintain engagement for more than a minute or so.

As we learned from the horses, sometimes you lose that connection and you have to pause, assess the horse's level of arousal through observing non-verbal cues from the horse and use the surge or rock back and sigh to energize or relax the horse as needed. By working on your own coherence and intention, you can see when the connection is restored. This continual sensitivity to someone else's level of focus and arousal, and ability to bring back their attention using your own self-regulation is critical in sustaining a meaningful connection.

HOW HORSES CAN STIMULATE SOCIAL CONNECTION

As people become more aware of their own body sensations and better able to observe the horse to understand what is being communicated to them, the horse and person can engage in a two-way conversation, which in time may result in social bonding. During my research, I have noticed that participants who bond with their horse are eager to share their experience with others, encouraging social interaction. This was particularly evident during our study at Hacienda at the River senior living community in Tucson, Arizona, which has an on-site equine program (Baldwin et al. 2021). Twenty-four residents and associates, aged

55 or over (but mostly over 70), consented to physiological measurements before, during and after four guided sessions of stroking one of three horses for ten minutes over four to six weeks.

During the exit interviews after their interaction with the horse, participants reported increased feelings of connection to the horse. They used words such as "connection," "bonding," "relaxed" and "calm." The experience also encouraged them to socially engage with the other participants and with the researchers. The degree of social interaction we observed throughout each session increased during the later weeks of the study. Many people in their 80s, 90s and over are not used to identifying their personal feelings and speaking about them. The fact that they became more willing to speak with the research assistants about their sensual experiences with the horses indicates that they were becoming more aware of their bodily sensations and less inhibited. These benefits of EAL for the elderly are illustrated in the following case study.

CASE STUDY: Heart breath and stroking – how a horse facilitates social bonding
Ann L. Baldwin, PhD, Physiologist, HeartMath Certified Trainer, Usui Reiki Master, Mind-Body-Science (abaldwin@mind-body-science.com)

PN had just moved into an assisted living community, Hacienda at the River, which ran an EAL program called "In the Presence of Horses." Her children had had their own ponies when they were small and so she was familiar with horses. To implement the EAL program at Hacienda at the River, specially trained and selected horses are trailered in three mornings a week so that the residents can interact with them under the guidance of equine professionals. PN, who was in her 80s, had been a "corporate wife" whose roles included piloting her husband's company plane and raising three children. She was now in the early stages of dementia and was becoming more and more withdrawn, barely speaking.

On PN's move-in day, one daughter brought her to the horses for her first EAL session. Emphatically, PN said that she was coming to the horses every day they were on site, Tuesday, Wednesday and Thursday. Later, the other daughter, who was supervising the move-in, visited to see how her mother and sister were faring with the horses. She remarked that seeing her mother so talkative, actively engaged and relating to both horses and horse staff felt surreal to her; nobody in the family had seen or heard their mother vocally and socially interacting for at least two years. Both sisters left for lunch with their mother saying they felt they "had their mother back."

A collaborative partnership between the EAL program and the University of Arizona was in place at that time to objectively study the degree to which stroking the horses, while breathing more slowly and deeply than usual, affects the residents' tendency to socially interact. PN consented to participate in this study. The on-site equine accommodation was situated in the front of the main building on a busy road and so it was not particularly quiet. The accommodation consisted of a purpose-built 20-by-30-foot equine paddock with covered porch and special equine pavers (non-slip, well drained, suitable for walkers, canes and wheelchairs), cooled main room, office and ADA-compliant bathroom. There was a selection of four facilitators and two equine professionals, trained in CPR and first aid, all solid in their horse–human interaction skills.

During the study, PN was directed as follows:

- Please focus your attention on the area of your heart.
- As you breathe in, imagine the breath going into your heart. As you breathe out, imagine the breath is leaving your heart.
- Count slowly to five as you breathe in and slowly to five as you breathe out. One and two and three and four and five.
- Now direct your breath heart beam towards the horses and sense/feel which horse's heart is calling to your heart.
- As you breathe in, imagine the breath is coming from the THAT horse's heart to your heart. As you breathe out, imagine your breath is going from YOUR heart to your chosen horse's heart.

At that point, PN selected her horse. The participants usually selected the horse that was showing the most interest in them; the signal may be a look, a movement of the head, an ear cocked in their direction or an actual approach, walking toward the participant who is sending breath heart beams. The participant approached the horse in greeting, arm outstretched, palm down. Once the horse looked at the participant or turned an ear towards them, the participant continued their approach to step forward and stroke the horse gently with one or both hands for 10–15 minutes. Participants were encouraged to be silent and focus on their breath and sensations. Afterwards, each participant was interviewed and asked to describe what sensations they felt in their body during the interactions. PN selected a horse named Joe for all four consecutive sessions that were included in the study.

PN, like most of the participants, showed an improvement in mood after her interactions with the horse and reported increased feelings of connection to the horse. The interns who analyzed the behavioral reports and exit interviews reported that PN became more attentive and vocal from week one to four, and her responses changed from short, clipped statements to more wordy, descriptive answers. Common "feeling" words she used in her exit interviews included "connection," "bond," "relaxed" and "calm." PN also became more expressive and showed more social engagement with the facilitator and interns as her time in the study increased.

How did this happen? Deep, slow exhales as we breathe stimulate the ventral vagus nerve. When we touch or are touched, that contact stimulates sensors below the skin that also signal the brain to stimulate the vagus nerve. According to the polyvagal theory, the ventral branch of the vagus nerve serves the muscles that control facial expression, speaking, swallowing and making eye contact, which all contribute to promoting social engagement. In addition, gentle touch can cause release of oxytocin, a neuropeptide that promotes feelings of trust and bonding. So, it was not surprising that PN experienced release from her self-induced social isolation after interacting with the horses in this way.

Apart from behavioral changes, PN showed a physiological shift in her HRV, as did most of the other participants. The frequency at which her heart rate was varying, or oscillating, when she stroked the horse exactly matched that of the horse, within an accuracy of three decimal points. Prior to the interaction, the HRV frequencies of PN and Joe were different from each other. This synchronization of HRV frequencies occurred during all four of her interactions with Joe that were measured. Coupling of HRV oscillation frequencies between horses and humans has been noted previously (Lanata *et al.* 2016). Those authors hypothesized that "human and horse can be considered as two complex systems, and when they are in visual, olfactory or physical contact they get interacting through a coupling process."

Another group has hypothesized that when a horse and a human experience a cardiovascular coupling during an interaction, there is also mutual coordination of emotional states (Scopa *et al.* 2020). So,

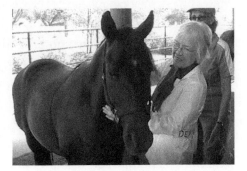

FIGURE 8.5 PN AND JOE.

the fact that PN and Joe consistently showed coupling of their HRV oscillations suggests not only that bonding was occurring between them on an emotional or behavioral level but that it was also manifesting physiologically.

PN proved to be a reliable regular EAL participant. She began to help co-teach the other residents as they moved in and visited the stables for their horse interactions. She was especially adept at teaching safety around the horses in the small, covered porch area, demonstrating the best way to approach a horse waiting to be greeted. A photo of PN with Joe is shown in Figure 8.5.

NEUROCEPTION OF SAFETY BY HORSE AND HUMAN: THE POLYVAGAL THEORY

As described in Chapter 7, according to the polyvagal theory, there are three distinct autonomic states, sympathetic hyperarousal or "fight or flight," parasympathetic hyperarousal, in which the dorsal vagus nerve is so highly stimulated by fear that one becomes immobilized (the freeze response), and ventral vagal activation which brings with it a state of "relaxed alertness," a feeling of safety and propensity for social engagement. Of course, these states are part of a whole spectrum of ANS responses in which sympathetic, dorsal vagal and ventral vagal systems are activated to varying degrees in any given moment.

Most people shift throughout the spectrum during their day, rarely reaching full-scale sympathetic or dorsal vagal stimulation. They use their power of neuroception to varying degrees to identify where they are on the ANS spectrum and to alter their behavior if necessary – for example, if it is clearly inappropriate and will not benefit themselves or others. However, trauma can shift the ANS into a state of sympathetic hyperarousal ("fight or flight" response) or, in severe cases, into a dorsal vagal freeze response. People suffering from trauma can get stuck in these states unless they can rebalance the ANS by stimulating the ventral vagal complex.

As explained in Chapter 7, somatic therapy uses techniques such as body awareness, body scanning and grounding while focusing on regulation of the breath. These techniques are frequently used with clients by EAL facilitators to provide a feeling of safety and security with the horses. Learning and growth cannot happen in an unsafe space. In return, the horses provide feedback to the client by altering their behavior, ranging from perhaps an inclination of an ear towards the client to a soft whisper of their breath on the client's cheek. These reactions sometimes profoundly affect the client, giving them a renewed sense of confidence and trust, as illustrated in the following case study.

CASE STUDY: Healing trauma by connecting with a horse

Linda Kohanov, Author, Founder, Coach and Teacher of
techniques using healing potential of horse–human relationships,
Eponaquest Worldwide (rasa@eponaquest.com)

When Margaret attended her first workshop at Eponaquest in Amado, AZ, she had endured several years of painful events that reawakened childhood trauma not previously addressed. She was seeing a therapist and was looking for ways to move more efficiently to a state of physical, mental, emotional and spiritual health. She had no horse experience but had read my first book *The Tao of Equus: A Woman's Journey of Healing and Transformation through the Way of the Horse.* Despite her skeptical, scientifically trained mind, she found the idea of working with horses to be inexplicably (in her mind) intriguing.

Her urge to explore the healing potential of the horse–human bond was powerful and not at all convenient: she had to travel from her home base in Canada to my Arizona ranch in order to attend what turned out to be several years of workshops and private intensives. She eventually became an associate instructor in Eponaquest's leadership and personal development techniques and is incorporating some of the principles and techniques into professional development for the people who live and work in nursing homes, particularly those approaches related to activating the vagus nerve through breathing techniques. (These can be taught, to a certain extent, without having to bring horses into the context in which she works, though Margaret insists the horses are the master facilitators of these shifts.)

Margaret's trauma became pronounced in her 50s, which was surprising and disorienting for her. She noticed it mostly in terms of disconnected somatic experiences and disquiet, and in life decisions whose motivations she found difficult to access. After gaining a PhD, she had experienced much professional success in academic fields and research. She was also very athletic. However, later in life, childhood trauma memories were triggered by a number of medical procedures, including cancer surgery and treatment, and some invasive procedures that caused her significant pain in movement and made her unsteady on her feet. Cognitively, she developed a growing awareness that too much seemed to be "going wrong" given the robust physical health of her parents and grandparents and a relatively healthy lifestyle.

Margaret's demeanor during the first day of the Eponaquest workshop exemplified body language associated with dorsal vagal activation. Her facial expressions were bland, her voice was monotone, and she rarely made eye contact. She would often look down when speaking to the group. This flat affect was all the more striking when I learned that she was known as an accomplished international speaker and was an experienced supervisor of university research teams.

One of the first activities we teach during our workshops is what we call the "rock back and sigh." This involves mindfully approaching a loose horse and noticing when the horse shows body language that he is alert to the human's presence. The human is then taught to rock back slightly and sigh, which is a long, relaxed outbreath. We have noticed that unrestrained horses are attracted to people as they audibly exhale and have since learned that a long out-breath can activate the ventral vagal complex. Since the ventral vagus facilitates "safety through connection," it makes sense that the "rock back and sigh" technique would attract a loose horse. The ventral vagus is activated in the horse and human at that moment. Ann Baldwin and I also learned from various studies we collaborated on that a state of "coherence" is even more attractive to horses.

That first day, Margaret was amazed that a simple breathing technique employed at a distance could cause a 1000-pound horse to come to her and gently interact. She was thrilled, and deeply moved. Her tear-filled eyes were bright and excited. She was noticeably more engaged, first with the horse, then with me as facilitator, then with her workshop colleagues. She commented that she felt more open and relaxed yet still energized as she practiced the "rock back and sigh" technique and, later, the coherent breathing technique, with several different horses.

Over the course of the first workshop, she was able to deepen her connecting experiences with the horses and, with one of my black horses, able to experience a deep openness and attunement – what we understand as entrainment where she experienced his bigger, slower heartbeat as beating in her chest and, as she described it later, as healing filaments in the networks of her brain. Her therapist noticed the difference and encouraged her to continue with the horse-facilitated work.

Eventually, she learned how to use "breathing as a language" with the horses and with her students and patients. She became more fluid in her movements and steady on her feet. Now, when she attends or assists at my workshops, she immediately engages with people, and her natural wit and intelligence come through loud and clear. She still describes her early experiences as vivid and very much present for her, none more so than the experience of entrainment and with it, a peace and stillness – states she still does not encounter easily without the support of the horses.

EPILOGUE

According to the Professional Association of Therapeutic Horsemanship, as of December 31, 2018, there were 873 centers with 4776 certified professionals and 61,642 volunteers working in these centers. Equine Assisted Learning is a growing industry and so these figures are underestimates of the current situation. An overview of facilities that engage in training, apprenticeship, internship and certification programs in EAL worldwide can be found at: https://equusoma. com/wp-content/uploads/2018/10/List-of-Equine-Assisted-Practice-Train-ings-and-Certifications-September-2018.pdf.

Although the field of EAL is rapidly growing, not everybody may have access to an EAL center or a certified practitioner. For that reason, many people ask, "Why horses? Won't some other animal do?" The answer is no. Although there is some evidence that pets such as dogs can improve your mood and reduce your blood pressure, especially when you stroke them, the findings are inconsistent (Schreiner 2016). Heart rate variability has improved, worsened or remained the same in the limited number of studies considering companion animals. In addition, the results of these studies may depend on the degree of bonding of the owner with the animal, usually a dog. On the other hand, nearly all the humans who interacted with horses in the research studies described in this chapter experienced a significant increase in HRV even though they were not familiar with the horses.

There is another reason for using horses rather than dogs in this type of work. Based on personal observations by myself and my colleagues, dogs tend to offer unconditional affection, especially to their owners if kept under favorable conditions, whereas horses usually require one to try to acknowledge and release any felt tension to some degree before they will engage. In this way, horses are good teachers for people who wish to improve their skills at stimulating their ventral vagal complex.

Whether or not you are able to experience EAL, practicing some of the exercises described in this book, either alone or with others, will greatly enrich your life and improve your physical, mental and emotional health. To help you with these goals, an appendix is provided, following this chapter, that includes summaries of the various exercises, as well as routines for using combinations of exercises on a daily, weekly and monthly basis.

REFERENCES

Baldwin AL, Rector BK and Alden AC, 2018. Effects of a form of equine-facilitated learning on heart rate variability, immune function, and self-esteem in older adults. *People and Animals: The International Journal of Research and Practice*. 1(1): Article 5.

Baldwin AL, Rector R and Alden AC, 2021. Physiological and behavioral benefits for people and horses during guided interactions at an assisted living residence. *Behavioral Sciences*. 11(10): 129. doi: 10.3390/bs11100129.

Baldwin AL, Walters L, Rector BK and Alden AC. 2023. Effects of equine interaction on mutual autonomic nervous system responses and interoception in a learning program for older adults. *People and Animals: The International Journal of Research and Practice*. 6(1): Article 3.

Brämer D, Günther A, Rupprecht S *et al.,* 2019. Very low frequency heart rate variability predicts the development of post-stroke infections. *Transl Stroke Res*. 10: 607–619. doi: 10.1007/s12975-018-0684-1.

Lampert R, Bremner JD, Su S *et al.,* 2008. Decreased heart rate variability is associated with higher levels of inflammation in middle-aged men. *Am Heart J*. 156(4): 759.e1–7. doi: 10.1016/j.ahj.2008.07.009.

Lanata A, Guidi A, Valenza G *et al.,* 2016. Quantitative heartbeat coupling measures in human-horse interaction. *Annu Int Conf IEEE Eng Med Biol Soc*. 2016: 2696–2699.

Ryan ML, Ogilvie MP, Pereira BMT *et al.,* 2011. Heart rate variability is an independent predictor of morbidity and mortality in hemodynamically stable trauma patients. *The Journal of Trauma: Injury, Infection, and Critical Care*. 7(6): 1371–1380. doi: 10.1097/TA.0b013e31821858e6.

Schreiner PJ, 2016. Emerging cardiovascular risk research: impact of pets on cardiovascular risk prevention. *Curr Cardiovasc Risk Rep*. 10(2): 8. doi: 10.1007/s12170-016-0489-2.

Scopa C, Greco A, Contalbrigo L *et al.,* 2020. Inside the interaction: contact with familiar humans modulates heart rate variability in horses. *Front Vet Sci*. 7: 582759. doi: 10.3389/fvets.2020.582759.

Shah A J, Lampert R, Goldberg J *et al.,* 2013. Posttraumatic stress disorder and impaired autonomic modulation in male twins. *Biol Psychiatry*. 73(11): 1103–1110. doi: 10.1016/j.biopsych.2013.01.019.

Stein PK, Barzilay JI, Chaves PH *et al.,* 2008. Higher levels of inflammation factors and greater insulin resistance are independently associated with higher heart rate and lower heart rate variability in normoglycemic older individuals: the Cardiovascular Health Study. *J Am Geriatr Soc*. 56(2): 315–321. doi: 10.1111/j.1532-5415.2007.01564.x.

Summary of Exercises to Activate the Ventral Vagus Complex

These are exercises you can do by yourself without any special equipment or practitioner.

Lavender aromatherapy (Chapter 2)

Buy a high-quality lavender essential oil and add a few drops to the water in a diffuser. Sit or lie down comfortably and breathe slowly as you smell the lavender vapor.

Om chant (Chapter 3)

Breathe in normally and say "Om" while exhaling. There should be definite pronunciation of each of the syllables, "A," "U" and "M," with a gradual transition of one to another. "A" is pronounced as "a" in "palm," "U" is pronounced as "ooo," and "M" is pronounced as a humming sound by closing the lips "mmmmmmm." The sound of "A" should start at the navel, "U" from the chest and "M" from brain (head).

Touch lips (Chapter 4)

Just run your fingers lightly over your lips to stimulate these vagal nerve endings. It is an easy way to relax.

Heart-Focused Breathing™ (HFB) (Chapters 4, 5)

Focus on your heart or chest area as you breathe, imagining the breath entering and leaving your heart, while breathing slightly more deeply and slowly than usual. Consciously relax all your muscles on every exhale.

Quick Coherence™ (Chapters 4, 8)

Start with HFB and then breathe in a "heart feeling," imagining a simple experience that brings warm feelings of genuine appreciation and gratitude in your heart.

Walking in nature (Chapter 4)

Walk in green areas, near trees and water, for 15–30 minutes twice a week.

Gassho breathing (modified for non-Reiki practitioners) (Chapter 5)

Concentrate on breathing in and out slowly through your nose (about five seconds in and five seconds out). With each in-breath, imagine that a beam of light is entering your crown and filling your entire body. With each out-breath, visualize that you are exhaling light from every pore in your body and off out to infinity.

Mindfulness eating (Chapter 6)

Eat a small piece of food and chew very slowly, while paying close attention to the actual sensory experience of eating: the sensations and movements of chewing, the flavor of the food as it changes, and the sensations of swallowing. Just pay attention, moment by moment.

Body awareness: first step of body scan (Chapter 7)

Recognize and identify areas of tension in the body, as well as calming thoughts and feelings.

Body scan (Chapter 7)

Find a quiet space where you can sit or lie down comfortably for some time between five and 30 minutes. Gradually sense the feelings in your body starting with your feet and ending with your neck, face and head. If you notice any areas of tension, pause to mindfully attend to this tension, then deliberately allow it to dissipate and release. Maintain a focus on the rhythm of your breath as you slowly breathe in and out, allowing any physical discomfort to be released as you exhale.

Orientation (Chapter 7)

After settling down, either sitting or standing, let your eyes and senses gently scan the environment. Notice an object, a color or a shape of particular interest. Let your senses rest there for a bit and let your eyes and whole body "receive" rather than "retrieve." Sit back and receive the sense of your environment. Notice your body and breath. You may experience ease, quietude, softness, fullness or centeredness.

Exercises that fit well together

1. HFB, Quick Coherence with lavender aromatherapy.
2. Touch lips, mindfulness eating.
3. HFB while forest bathing.
4. Om chant while forest bathing.
5. Touch lips, body awareness, body scan.
6. Orientation, touch lips, Om chant.
7. Lavender aromatherapy, body awareness, Gassho breathing.

Suggested routines for exercises and therapies

- **Daily:** HFB, Quick Coherence, Gassho breathing, touch lips, aromatherapy, body awareness, body scan, Om chant.
- **Weekly:** Laughter yoga, breath-focused yoga, singing group, mindfulness eating, eating with friends, Om chant, body scan, forest bathing, orientation.
- **Monthly:** Auricular acupuncture, massage (with neck and shoulder emphasis), Equine Assisted Learning, colon hydrotherapy (especially for non-inflammatory bowel discomfort), somatic therapy (especially for anxiety, stress, chronic pain).

Subject Index

Note: Page numbers to figures (f), tables (t) and boxes (b) are given in italics

Author Index